PRIMARY CARE DE

# Future Options for General Practice

### Edited by **Geoff Meads**
Director of Performance Management,
South and West Regional Health Authority

Foreword by **Ian Carruthers**
Chief Executive
Dorset Health Authority

Series Editors **Pat Gordon** and **Diane Plamping**

Published in association with King's Fund, London

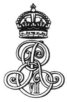

**Radcliffe Medical Press**
Oxford and New York

Radcliffe Medical Press Ltd
18 Marcham Road, Abingdon, Oxon OX14 1AA, UK

Radcliffe Medical Press, Inc.
141 Fifth Avenue, New York, NY 10010, USA

British Library Cataloguing in Publication Data

A catalogue record for this book is available from the British Library.


ISBN 1 85775 079 9


Library of Congress Cataloging-in-Publication Data
Future options for general practice: primary care development/edited by
Geoff Meads; foreword by Ian Carruthers.
    p. cm.
  Includes bibliographical references and index.
  Other title: Primary care development.
  ISBN 1-85775-079-9
  1. Primary care (Medicine)—Practice—Great Britain. I. Meads, Geoff.
  [DNLM: 1. Family Practice—trends—Great Britain. 2. Primary Health
Care—trends—Great Britain.   W 89 F9965 1995]
R729.5.G4F88 1995
362.1′0941—dc20
DNLM/DLC
for Library of Congress
                                                              95-23235
                                                                   CIP

Typeset by AMA Graphics Ltd, Preston
Printed and bound in Great Britain

# Contents

# Contributors

Stuart Chidgey, Independent Consultant in Primary Care, Praed Consulting, The Medical Centre, Abbotsham Road, Bideford, Devon, EX39 3AF

David Colin-Thomé, General Practitioner, Health Centre, Chester Close, Castlefields, Runcorn, WA7 2HY

Tom Davies, General Practitioner, Health Centre, Landsdowne Road, Yaxley, Peterborough, PE7 3JL

Roger Edmonds, General Practitioner, former Chairman, Wessex General Practice Advisory Committee, 11 Salisbury Road, Andover, Hampshire, SP10 2JJ

John Horder, General Practitioner, former President, Royal College of General Practitioners, 98 Regent's Park Road, London, NW1 8UG

June Huntington, Independent Consultant in Primary Care, 23 Daleham Gardens, London, NW3 6BY

John Hughes, General Practitioner, Havant Health Centre, Suite B, Civic Centre Road, Havant, Hampshire, PO9 2AQ

Hugh Maclean, General Practitioner, Fleming House, 92 Carisbrooke Road, Newport, Isle of Wight, PO30 1DE

Geoff Meads, Director of Performance Management, South and West Regional Health Authority, Westward House, Lime Kiln Close, Stoke Gifford, Bristol, BS12 6SR

David Paynton, General Practitioner, Health Centre, Commercial Street, Bitterne, Southampton

Patrick Pietroni, General Practitioner and Professor of Community Care and Primary Health University of Westminster, 33 Queen Anne Street, London, W1M 9FB

Barry Robinson, General Practitioner, Lyme Community Care Centre, Uplyme Road, Lyme Regis, Dorset, DT7 3LS

Robert Sloane, Chief Executive, Andover Community Health Services Trust, Charlton Road, Andover, Hampshire, SP10 3LB

Nigel Starey, General Practitioner and Medical Advisor, North West Anglia Health Commission, St John's, Thorpe Road, Peterborough, PE3 6JG

Nigel Sylvester, General Practitioner, Friarsgate Health Centre, Winchester, Hampshire, SO23 8EF

# Series introduction

Primary care development is arguably the most important topic for the NHS to get to grips with in the rapidly changing environment of the 1990s. This new series of books about primary care development is intended to be topical, useful and, before very long, out-of-date. It is based on the current work of the King's Fund Primary Care Group and the ideas, experience and inspiration of a number of people who have worked with us and shared their enthusiasms.

Primary care is often used to mean general practice. Here it is used in the broader sense to include the network of community-based health services which in the UK allow us to manage 90% of care outside hospitals; to manage earlier, safer discharge from hospitals, and to maintain people at home who do not want to be institutionalized.

From a position of relative neglect and invisibility, primary care has shot to the top of the NHS policy agenda. This has much to do with the NHS reforms and the drive to control public spending. Like all industrialized nations faced with ever-increasing costs in health care, we are experimenting with reorganization. Since hospitals use most NHS resources, this is where most attention was directed and primary care became the focus only as a potentially cheaper option. But the drive for efficiency and value for money coincides with other powerful influences which challenge us to examine alternatives to traditional ways of delivering services. If effective primary care really is the key to successful health services in the future, then recognizing its distinctive characteristics, and what we value about it as well as what we want to change becomes critical. In other words, primary care has development needs in its own right quite apart form the current emphasis on the shift from secondary to primary care – the so-called substitution agenda.

This new series is about ideas and services which are being developed and tested around the country. Geoff Meads' book *Future Options for General Practice* describes a number of experimental working models of primary care organizations. The names they are given may still be provisional at this time but the message for the future is clear. Partnership is no longer the only option. There are new ways of delivering practice-based primary care. Some will be replicated. Others are probably unique. They are developing in a period which is seen by some GPs to offer maximum opportunity for experiment while, paradoxically, others see little but damage and dismay.

Other titles in the series address the potential conflict in values between practices and their practitioners, new ways of extending primary care beyond family-based practice, and practice management – the fastest growing health care occupation in the UK.

We hope the ideas in these books contribute to the debate about the future shape of the NHS and are useful to the people working in the middle of these major changes now.

Pat Gordon
King's Fund
London

October 1995

# Foreword

Primary care is becoming the principal focus for health and health services delivery throughout the National Health Service and the NHS Executive's publication of *Towards a Primary Care Led NHS* in October 1994 represented a further watershed in the development of primary care to the year 2000 and beyond. We can now look forward to many challenges as we all strive to improve local health and patient services, with general practice increasingly becoming the focus for these activities.

In order to take advantage of the opportunities that lie ahead in these challenges, it is essential that full support and encouragement is given to developing stronger organizations to purchase and provide health and social care in primary care settings.

The development of a varied range of primary care organizations has already begun and this text presents an excellent summary to date in this increasingly important area.

*Future Options for General Practice* is essential reading for everybody engaged in health care. I believe its thought provoking contributions will provide a catalyst for the future development of primary care and the delivery of better local health services for our communities.

Ian Carruthers
Yeovil, 18 May 1995

# Preface

By 1 April 1996 about 100 new Health Authorities will have completed their 'shadow' period and come into full legislative force. Merging the functions of DHAs and FHSAs they are charged with commissioning the best value for health and health care. For the first time virtually all NHS resources will be at their disposal. How will they deploy the combined financial allocations for primary and secondary care to support their new capacity to enter into local contracts? Which health care providers will emerge in this market place in response to this shift in new commissioning power?

For general practice these are critical questions. New Authorities will want to invest more in primary care but not necessarily in the conventional manner. The traditional model of general practice based on the independent contractor has already been threatened by the advent of fundholding. The monopoly protection afforded by a national General Medical Services contract will become much less secure as new Health Authorities draft their own services agreements to supplement or even, over time, to replace 'The Red Book'.

This publication defines some of the future options for the future organization of primary care. It starts from the assumption that while the orthodox legal partnership of a group practice is robust enough to survive in the UK, where there is a deep rooted attachment to the GPs professional leadership of primary care, it will rapidly become only one of a number of provider options. There will be neither a right nor a wrong form of organization. Local circumstances will increasingly be the key determinant of what is required to achieve equivalent services and outcomes to respond to a particular community's needs.

Many, perhaps most, of the organizational initiatives will come from GPs themselves. Some will come from their potential competitors. A few may emerge from the new Health Authorities, especially where required by the past neglect of primary care services development. Others will develop as a result of the extensions to fundholding.

This book reflects this mixture. Written largely by GPs for GPs, it also, for example, includes ideas and initiatives which will be of real value to managers reconfiguring NHS Community Trusts and professionals looking at how they address the challenges of substitution. It is a book for the planners, providers and purchasers of extended primary care, whether in the public or independent sectors. The NHS reforms have been a voyage of discovery. The following chapters help steer a course.

Much of this book is about teamwork and the opportunities for its expression in primary care. One such team was the Wessex Regional Health Authority's Primary Care Directorate from 1992 to 1994. Alison Smithies, Elizabeth Sibley, Andrew Cawthron, Ian Allured and Kevan Kenny, in particular, will recognize in this book several of the developments they helped to stimulate. I am grateful for their support and for that of their mentor June Huntington whose concluding chapter characteristically makes sense of what is an increasingly diffuse subject. I am also grateful to Rennie Fritchie and Ian Carruthers, the leadership of the new South and West Regional Health Authority, for sustaining an environment, in the aftermath of Wessex, which continues to stimulate creative thought and action. Finally, I must thank Jane Harding whose precision in preparing the manuscript has been matched by her much tested patience.

The book is dedicated to Sarah our first born which, given the new ground covered by its content, feels appropriate.

Geoff Meads
Winchester

April 1995

*To Sarah*

# Abbreviations

| | |
|---|---|
| CHC | Community Health Council |
| CMHT | Community Mental Health Team |
| DHA | District Health Authority |
| FHSA | Family Health Services Authority |
| GMSC | General Medical Services Committee |
| GMS | General Medical Services |
| GP | General practitioner |
| GPFH | General practice fundholding |
| HCHS | Hospital and Community Health Services |
| IMT | Information management and technology |
| IT | Information technology |
| NHS | National Health Service |
| NHSE | National Health Service Executive |
| PCLP | Primary care led purchasing |
| PCT | Primary Care Team |
| PFI | Private Finance Initiative |
| PHCT | Primary Health Care Team |
| RCGP | Royal College of General Practitioners |
| RHA | Regional Heath Authority |
| SSD | Social Services Department |
| UK | United Kingdom |
| VTS | Vocational Training Scheme |
| WHO | World Health Organization |

# The British dilemma   1

*Geoff Meads*

## General practice: principle and organization

The 1990s have been years of unprecedented change in health and health care systems throughout the developed world. Yet, even against this background, the scale and pace of change in the UK stands out. In less than five years, all secondary health care services will have been converted into National Health Service (NHS) Trusts; Health Authorities reduced in number by two-thirds to around 100 (with a parallel reduction in waiting times); and general practice fundholding introduced to half the population with an overall financial allocation in excess of £4 billion. By April 1996, the first statutory NHS bodies dedicated to the managed development of primary care (the Family Health Services Authorities (FHSAs)) will have closed. From April 1996, primary care will lead the management and development of the NHS.

The impact of the combined policies represented by *The patient's charter*[1], the *Health of the nation strategy*[2] and the implementation of the *Working for patients* White Paper[3] has been immense. Yet, even in this revolutionary period when the maintenance of some of the founding values of the NHS has been questioned, the principle of general practice has never been challenged. Such is the deep-rooted public confidence in general practice that national policy adjustments to it, as a basic principle, remain inconceivable. Indeed, at a time when the NHS is being criticized for its alleged shift away from its traditional obligations of ensuring free and equal access to comprehensive care, the central reliance on general practice as the constant expression of this responsibility has grown. Accordingly, as a principle, it is being reinvented by the new Health Authorities in their strategies for monitoring and supporting a primary care led NHS[4] from April 1996.

Table 1.1 provides a typical example of the local approaches being adopted. This illustration from East Sussex[5], also indicates how the principle of general practice is no longer simply being attached to a single individual. The association now is with a number of professionals equipped to undertake a generalist role. The role remains continuing personal care, but its components and contributors are changing. With primary care having to absorb and respond to both providing and commissioning roles (the separation of which was at the heart of the original NHS reforms in 1991) general practice as principle and organization is no longer one. As the following chapters demonstrate, the preservation of the principle is requiring the rapid development of general practices as very different kinds of local primary care organizations throughout the UK.

# From strategic planning to local participation

That such changes are now able to take place signals a basic change in the developmental framework of the NHS; it is becoming a complex of local health care markets. The European standard of subsidiarity now holds sway in terms of

**Table 1.1** What do we mean by primary care?

*Primary care is easier to describe than to define, but it has the following characteristics*

- It is **first contact care**, hence the name

- It is readily accessible by **self-referral**

- It is provided in a **home** or **community setting**

- It is **comprehensive** and **holistic**, from **cradle** to **grave** (or even earlier with pre-conceptual and antenatal care), and grounded in a **social** and **family context**

- It is led by professionals who have trained for a **generalist** role

- It is **continuing** and **personal** care and the **fixed point** for those tapping in to wider networks of social or hospital care

- It is increasingly capable of providing acute care, high-technology care and specialist care, and **referrals between one primary care professional and another** are an increasing trend

- Primary care has at its core a large number of **independent contractors**, working in **teams** with directly employed practice staff and employees of **NHS Trusts**, with links into the **voluntary, statutory** and **private sectors**

- Above all, it is deeply entrenched in the **culture** and **tradition** of health care in this country, **cherished** by those who use it

maximizing local decision-making powers. Before 1991, NHS strategic planning was based on a combination of professional norms, public health data and capital project proposals and plans were made for 10-year periods. This system is now redundant and in its place is an NHS developmental process which is essentially participative and increasingly political in its local expression.

The central NHS strategic framework has already reduced annual planning priorities to single figures and gives abundant licence for local initiative and innovation. Primary care has become the NHS laboratory for experimentation, for the trial and error 'learning by doing' approaches that come with a readily reversible annual contracting cycle. 'Bolt on' practice-based agreements, augmenting the nationally negotiated General Medical Services (GMS) contract and covering such services as chiropody and physiotherapy, were initiated by such frontiers as Cambridgeshire FHSA and Dorset District Health Authority (DHA) in 1990/1. They have now become widespread wherever purchasing Health Commissions have been created to combine primary and secondary care funding. NHS Community Health Services Trusts have wooed their local practices (and potential purchasing proprietors), with outposted consultant clinics in specialisms ranging from dermatology to child psychiatry. Community hospitals are increasingly coming under the supervision of local general practices. Sometimes they provide an alternative venue for out-of-hours services to the neighbourhood surgery. The physical limitations of neighbourhood surgeries as modern primary care centres are increasingly being addressed through new sources of private capital finance, such as major retail pharmacies and private insurers, who are keen to secure their market share as NHS downward pressure on prescribing expenditure and waiting lists begins to bite.

In short, primary care in the NHS is up for grabs. A development process which deliberately permits parallel track initiatives, duplication and issues central management guidance that explicitly encourages a competitive solution to virtually all market management issues[6], is one in which weaker practices will go to the wall and a new variety of stronger primary care organizations will emerge. As the following chapters illustrate, a provider market in primary care is beckoning which, by 1997/8 when they are established and secure, new Health Authorities should be ideally placed to exploit.

American-style managed care organizational arrange-ments, customized to the UK general practice scene, could well become the norm. Population units of 50–100 000 would be the standard basis for allocations, contracting and protocol-based services arranged across traditional primary and second-ary care settings and skill mixes[7]. Forward thinking GPs, like John Hughes (see Chapter 3), clearly recognize the importance of their profession taking control of the type of organizational development these commissioning units require, if GPs are to retain their sense of autonomy and control their own destinies. Nigel Sylvester's description of some future general practices as 'preferred providers' (see page 79) is a direct crib from the Minneapolis-inspired Health Maintenance Organizations' development of such health service units, with their compre-hensive range of primary and secondary care clinicians and internal gate-keeping mechanisms between the two[8].

Individual business plans are replacing overall strategic plans in the NHS development process. Organizational development in primary care for more effective health services increasingly means gaining a competitive edge as well as im-proved organizational viability.

## Primary care led purchasing

Primary care led purchasing (PCLP) was one of the products of the Wessex Regional Health Authority's commitment in 1991 to making 'primary care the principal focus of responsi-bility for health'[9]. As the RHA's subsequent market research showed this objective (one of eight) quickly became the most readily identifiable and was supported by local NHS employees and external agencies. Implementation involved wide-ranging initiatives, including dedicated capital, research and manage-ment development programmes, and the sponsorship of a plethora of service developments based in local general prac-tices. Above all, it entailed driving the joint resources of 15

**Table 1.2**   Wessex strategic framework

*The five main objectives*

• Practice-based primary care to be the preferred setting of services, wherever this is appropriate and effective for patients, and an efficient use of resources

• Extended practice-based primary care team services to be responsible for meeting the health needs of the majority of the population

• Practice-based contracts for primary care services to be the local responsibility of Health Commissions

• Primary care led purchasing to be the guiding principle to apply in meeting and responding to a population's needs

• Participation of the public to be a right throughout the planning, delivery and assessment of primary care

DHAs and FHSAs towards primary care development through their unified management by six Health Commissions.

By the end of 1994 much of the Wessex approach had been adopted nationwide, including PCLP. The meaning of this term, however, had become something quite different.

For Wessex, PCLP was one element in a five point regional framework for primary care development (Table 1.2), which was applied by each Health Commission over the period 1992–1994. PCLP was an important element, but not the most important. The simple framework emerged with widespread professional, managerial and member support through a series of workshops and learning events over 2 years, which clearly put the emphasis on the need to address the quality and range of primary care service provision. Sound general practice in both clinical and managerial terms was regarded as the qualifying prerequisite for PCLP.

This order of priorities, because of the consensus it attracted, served as a stimulus to PCLP. Unlike many other parts of the UK, the primary care setting in Wessex became the first port of call for DHA service contracts and not simply the control mechanism for secondary care referrals and expenditure. In Dorset, for example, about 50% of dermatology and audiology services had transferred from hospital settings by 1994. In Southampton, the newly created Health Commission Director of Primary Care ensured that virtually all practices had direct and immediate access to local physiotherapy, counselling and chiropody specialisms. At the end of 1994, over 90% of the 500 general practices in Wessex were actively engaged in different forms of PCLP, and were collaborating with the local Health Commission.

By the beginning of 1994, general practices in Wessex had taken the lead in creating what could then be separated into 10 distinct strands of PCLP (Table 1.3)[10]. These models helped to create the environment in which the sixth wave extensions to general practice fundholding could be announced in October 1994[4]. These included the new total fundholding groups and the purchasing of community health services by small practice combinations with lists of over 3000 patients, signalling the co-option by national policy into fundholding of otherwise potentially deviant PCLP alternatives. The effect is to make fundholding the exclusive option. It has become synonymous with PCLP.

Table 1.3    Wessex primary care led purchasing models, 1993–1994

- Input from individual practices to purchasing decisions (eg pan-Portsmouth Locality Commissioning model)

- Input from groups of general practices representative of the Commission area to purchasing decisions (eg Southampton GP Advisory Committee)

- Combinations of local primary care health teams (PHCTs) coming together to influence purchasing decisions (eg Aldershot and Alton Locality Purchasing Groups)

**Table 1.3** *continued*

- Local PHCTs compiling individual health plans for submission to the Commission to influence purchasing decisions (eg Bridport and Verwood, Dorset)

- Combinations of local PHCTs compiling one health plan to influence purchasing decisions (eg Hythe, Waterside Health Plan)

- Individual PHCTs compiling a health plan and being allocated indicative budgets by the Commission, but with purchasing still undertaken by the Commission (eg North and West Wiltshire Purchasing Consortium)

- Combinations of local PHCTs compiling a health plan to influence purchasing decisions and bidding for contracts for shared services (eg Swanage, Dorset)

- Individual PHCTs or groups of PHCTs compiling a local health plan and receiving allocations for the purchase and provision of agreed services (eg Isle of Wight General Practice Fundholding (GPFH) Consortium)

- Combinations of local PHCTs compiling a local health plan and social care plan and receiving allocations from the Commission for the purchase and provision of agreed services. Staff may be employed within the PHCTs as care managers with a limited budget for social care (eg Lyme Regis Community Care Unit, Dorset)

- Combinations of local PHCTs compiling a local health plan and social care plan and receiving allocations delegated by the Commission and Social Services Department for the purchase and provision of agreed services (eg Bath General Practices national pilot for PHCT/Community Mental Health Team (CMHT) development)

The effect in organizational terms has been to blur the separation of purchasing and providing functions which was the central platform of *Working for Patients*[3]. General practice is still a business, and one business. The business is primary patient care and, while the accounts may have to be separate, the monies that come from offering GMS and arranging hospital and community health services continue to go into a single pot to support this business.

However, the scale of the pooled resources is quite different from before. For an individual practice, it means managing £2 million rather than £200 000. As our surveys in Wessex over the 1992–1994 period show[11], it has meant a sudden influx into primary care of new skills and new roles, often drawn from personnel with banking, information management, insurance and general management backgrounds. It has meant NHS Community Trusts reorienting their services to individual practices and Health Authorities moving away from direct purchasing, as their role becomes that of advising commissioning general practices and supporting primary care in managing the increased demands that combining extended provider and purchasing functions entails.

The direction is that of larger organizations, different skill mixes and a conversion from independent contractor to independent sector status. The danger for both the NHS and individuals is that if this direction is built entirely on the fundholding version of PCLP it may distort the development of primary care and give undue priority to the purchasing element of its business. As both the Wessex PCLP experience and the following chapters in this book demonstrate, it remains essential that general practices are able to develop on their own local terms and always in (often different) ways that preserve and nurture the continuing personal care traditions and relationships of the primary care setting. In short, PCLP needs to be true to itself if alternative community based institutions are not simply to develop, relabelling people as 'patients' or worse 'consumers' or 'clients'.

# Integrating health and social services in primary care

Several of the following chapters suggest that this potential pitfall may be avoided by general practices absorbing what Professor Pietroni terms 'the discipline of community care' (*see* page 133), as their primary care organizations diversify and grow. While there is irony in general practitioners (GPs) embracing social workers (their traditional sparring partners) to ensure survival, there is also logic. Individual needs assessment applies equally now to the roots of care management and PCLP, and both entail devolving budgets and decision-making to the point closest to the individual in need. Accordingly, the integration of health and services in primary care has emerged as the key to development in the 1990s.

As PCLP developed more quickly in Wessex than elsewhere it has already become a significant trend in 1995. In Wiltshire and Somerset, there are 70 'Practice Linkworker' schemes at different stages of operation[12]. As the examples in Table 1.4 illustrate, these initiatives are largely about extending domiciliary support and rehabilitation services in an area where there is already an abundant supply of private residential and nursing homes. In other situations, where the latter are relatively scarce, often in or around major cities, as Patrick Pietroni (*see* Chapter 9) and Tom Davies (*see* Chapter 10) illustrate, extending the primary care team may mean encompassing the local hostel for disabled people or, as is already the case in Exeter and Cambridge, providing respite care facilities as an adjunct to a surgery or health centre.

This growing integration of health and social services in the primary care setting requires both health and local authority funding. It requires general practice businesses to contract into a further income stream: SSD's Service Local Agreements as traditionally applied to local voluntary groups and associations. Handicapped in the UK by the legacy of voluntary organizations being essentially lobby groups or representative

**Table 1.4**  Integrating health and social care: local examples in the South and West

*The main aim of integration has been to allow people a 'single door' access to both health and social care*

- GP linkworkers in Wiltshire and Bath Health Commission attached to 50% general practices in April 1995 and aiming for 75% coverage by April 1996, outcomes are:

  - effective bridging health and social services

  - effective commissioning of social care services for adult clients

  - provision of improved local user access to community care

- Somerset linkworker scheme has achieved similar benefits for service users as has an agreement with Social Services Department (SSD) whereby specialist district nurses have been made responsible for assessing older people's needs for nursing home care and have been able to access the necessary SSD budget to arrange appropriate placements (residential or at home with enhanced care)

- Joint commissioning for services provided in local community hospitals for older people based on locality planning groups with SSD, voluntary sector and user/carer representation with local GPs (Wiltshire and Bath). Outcome is increase in local services to meet the assessed needs of older people

- Purchase of nursing care by SSD care managers to enable people with a high level of nursing need to remain in their own homes (Dorset Health Commission). Such joint commissioning arrangements have:

  - improved understanding between health and social services

  - integrated arrangements to meet health and social care

**Table 1.4**  *continued*

---

- Provision of emergency and planned respite care in private residential and nursing homes via GPFH (Trowbridge) allowing immediate access to users and carers via either GP or social services with health and SSD each contributing half the costs. (Similar project started on Isle of Wight for elderly mentally frail people and their carers)
- Social worker for older people placed with GPFH practice on large estate in Basingstoke to:

  - provide integrated health and social care domiciliary packages

  - access and stimulate local voluntary sector activity

  - provide direct SSD input as required

All the above initiatives provide a local, co-ordinated and accessible route to integrated health and social care via primary care

---

bodies, such forward thinking authorities as Somerset and Hampshire have been only too pleased to contract with general practices, at a time when they are expected by central government to commit 85% of their £16.5 million (Somerset) and £52.1 million (Hampshire) to community care in the UK to independent sector, community-based providers in 1995/6. Obliged since 1991 to screen all their patients over 75 years annually, and increasingly responsible for how the funds attached to Community Health Services for people with special needs are deployed, the general practice is emerging as the arena in which the tension between longer life expectancy and earlier average disablement will be played out.

The implications for the organizational development of primary care arising from this convergence of health and social services are enormous. The new consortia of Health

Authorities formed on 1 April 1995 to commission non-medical education have, for example, quickly recognized the need for inter-professional programmes. By 1996, seven education establishments in the South and West NHS region, will be providing courses for forms of extended primary care team development. These range from Exeter and Plymouth Universities in the western peninsula to the Bournemouth University and Southampton Health Policy Institutes on the south coast. This geographical spread also applies to general practices that are following Barry Robinson's pioneering example in changing their names to community care centres, and his talent for attracting joint venture capital funding (*see* Chapter 13).

Whatever political changes lie ahead, it is hard to imagine general practices surrendering their move to fully fledged independent sector status, with its associated service and financial benefits. There can be no turning back the clock to pre-1990 GMS contract days and as the new 1996 Health Authorities gain confidence and the reformed unitary local authorities look to make their mark, further sound business opportunities for local negotiation are bound to arise.

## Summing up

What these trends amount to is the translation of PCLP to primary care led providing. With appropriate support, general practices are emerging as tomorrow's alternative providers. As the rest of this book argues, the exclusive legal partnership is an organizational arrangement that is too restricted to respond to the demands of this development in primary care. Other models are essential if the principle of general practice is to be sustained. With traditional NHS strategic planning being subsumed by increasingly local and participative processes for service development the task of keeping this goal in focus becomes even more difficult.

Nevertheless, this is a time of unprecedented opportunity for general practice, and for general practice based primary care. Ministerial policy and central management have never been so explicitly supportive. Resources are flowing one way. The inevitable reactions in terms of more strenuous performance monitoring and quality assurance have yet to come. In short, a window of opportunity exists for the practitioners to decide what the future options for general practice should be.

# References

1   Department of Health (1991) *The patient's charter.* HMSO, London.

2   Department of Health (1992) *The health of the nation: A strategy for health in England.* HMSO, London.

3   Department of Health (1989) *Working for patients.* HMSO, London.

4   Developing NHS purchasing and GP fundholding. (20 October 1994) EL (94) 79.

5   East Sussex Health Authority (February 1995) A strategy for the development of primary health care in East Sussex 1995–2000; Consultative Draft.

6   The operation of the NHS market: Local freedoms, National responsibilities. (12 December 1994) HSG (94) 55.

7   Nichol D (1995) *Next steps for purchasing? Population and personalised care management in best practice, in health care purchasing.* Churchill Livingstone, Edinburgh.

8   Hadley J P and Langwell K (1991) Managed care in the United States. *Health Policy.* **19**: 91–118.

9   Meads G (1993) RHAs and primary care: The new alliance. *Primary Care Management.* **3**: 2–4.

10  Based on Meads G (1995) All roads lead to ROME. In Henry S and Pickersgill D (eds) *Making sense of fundholding.* Radcliffe Medical Press, Oxford, p. 116.

11  Sibley E (1994) Preparing the leadership of tomorrow: An effective strategy for management development. *Primary Care Management.* **4**: 8–11.

12  Jones R (1995) Moving towards integrated health and social care management. *Primary Care Management.* **5**: 3–6.

# The international context    ⌐2

*John Horder*

It is easy and natural to think of primary care in the UK, its characteristics and development since the Second World War and the start of the NHS as an island story. It is the story of inherited traditions of general practice, district nursing and midwifery, forming elements in a coherent service. When the NHS started, it was possible rapidly to register almost the whole population with GPs. Over subsequent years the distribution of GPs throughout the country became even, compared with most other countries. Since some of them were already in partnership, the formation of groups of doctors, sharing premises, staff and equipment was easy. Other professionals became attached to the group and so the concept of 'the primary care team' emerged. Payment (mainly by capitation), lists of registered patients and case records which eventually covered the patient's life and moved if the person moved, all made a basis for including personal preventive activities in the remit of the primary care team. Overall, there was a steady increase in responsibilities, as these changes prepared general practice to cope with the stream of technical advances emerging from clinical and basic research. Research began, almost for the first time, to be undertaken within general practice itself. A specific postgraduate training was developed, along with the inclusion of general practice as a routine part of the training of medical students. All these developments, together with systematic efforts to raise quality, and improvements in the remuneration of GPs, changed primary care into the most attractive first choice of career for young doctors; a phenomenon unique among comparable countries during the same period.

If one feature in this story has been especially important, it has been the tradition of universal access to a generalist medical and nursing service, backed by specialist referrals, and by referral back. This has nearly eliminated direct access by patients to specialists for most problems. The tradition has been maintained in principle, and largely in practice, by patients, generalists and specialists alike, because each group has seen advantage in it. It has created an unusually clear distinction between two major elements in the health service. Against expectation, this has allowed the role of medical generalist to be developed and valued to an extent seen in only a few other countries, notably Denmark, the Netherlands and perhaps Canada.

We are used to the idea that the clinical practice of medicine is international. A clinical advance in one country is likely with little delay to change practice in other countries, especially specialist practice. Generalists have developed a little more slowly the means of exchanging clinical knowledge and skills across national boundaries; but these are now well established.

In contrast with clinical practice, there are good reasons for expecting that the organization of general practice or primary care will be nationally developed. It forms one element in a national health care system and such systems differ in form from one another. Moreover, primary care is influenced in each country by such distinctive elements in national, regional or local government as education, housing or communications.

In reality there have been international channels of communication for exchanging ideas about the organization of health care systems since 1945. International interest in the organization of general practice began to be seen in about 1960, notably in the World Health Organization (WHO), which appointed consultants and travelling Fellows with this focus of concern[1,2]. It was through this route, for example, that initial plans for the vocational training of GPs were influenced by a system of training already being implemented in Yugoslavia[3]. The linkage of primary care with population medicine and their joint application to the assessment of health needs owes much to the work of Kark in South Africa and Israel[4]. The attachment of nurses (and social workers) to GPs and the idea of a health team were partly stimulated from the USA by the Family Health Maintenance Demonstration[5,6]. More recent examples of ideas imported from that country have been the systematic development of quality assessment (performance review and audit), for instance in the work of Donabedian[7]; and the idea of an internal market in health care[8]. Much older and more fundamental examples of influence from other countries might be in the principle of sickness insurance, first introduced in Germany under Bismarck[9] or in the notion of paying doctors to keep people healthy (payment by capitation) attributed to a Chinese emperor long before Christ.

## The value of international exchange

The value of an international exchange of ideas depends on the degree to which the same problems are faced in different countries. This chapter concentrates on countries of comparable development, even though some lessons can be learned only from less developed countries, where basic problems stand out very clearly[10].

(A significant example is from Nigeria. An under-fives clinic, run by midwives under medical supervision, was established in one village, providing preventative and curative services. The children of another similar village, with minimal child-health services, served as controls. Both populations of children were observed for one year. The death rate in the first village was half that in the second[11].)

Comparisons will therefore be made and ideas sought from such countries as Denmark, France, Germany, the Netherlands, Sweden, Canada, USA, Japan, Singapore and Australia. (East European countries are too recently in transition.) How far then are general practice and primary care faced with the same problems and challenges in these countries and in others like them?

# Shared problems and challenges

Doctors and nurses in primary care in all these countries have to make at least initial responses to the needs of their people for technical and interpersonal care, for a wide range of conditions.

They all have to cope with a wide range of new knowledge and techniques applicable directly or by referral. They face individuals and populations with increasing knowledge of medicine and expectations that rise with every new development. People now seek increased participation in decision making and are increasingly ready to challenge professional authority, whether individually, through representative organizations or at the level of government.

## Demography, mortality, morbidity

Between the countries in question there are only small differences in the distribution of morbidity and in the main causes of death. They all experience an increase in the proportion of people of 65 and over 75 years of age. They have similar expectations of life, about 74 years for men and about 80 years for women[12]. In all of them, primary care deals increasingly with chronic illness, psychiatric illness, abuse of drugs and alcohol and with social problems.

The burden of rising expectations and increasing technical responsibilities has become an intrinsic problem in primary care. The number and variety of tasks, whether in prevention, assessment or management, that are now within the doctor's capability in primary care, are so great that sharing, delegation and teamwork have become unavoidable. However, these remedies themselves demand time and skills for communication and for education.

## Government intervention

Doctors and nurses in primary care in all these countries face governments and local administrations increasingly concerned about the increasing costs of health care. Costs are increasing due to rising expectations, new and expensive techniques and ageing populations requiring more care. Balancing costs and benefits is now a major concern in all these countries. Among them the UK is unusual in two ways: first, the percentage of national product devoted to health is very low compared with almost all of the other countries (*see* page 34, Appendix); second, the proportion of total health expenditure devoted to GMS (primary care) has been rising slowly for 15 years and is due to rise further if the present policy of transferring as much care as possible from secondary to primary sources is realized[13].

In most countries, the effect of government intervention in limiting resources has been felt more severely by those who work in hospitals. Direct or indirect control of primary care is more variable, but everywhere tends to increase. This is resented and initially resisted by professionals, accustomed to take pride (and sometimes advantage) in the international tradition of professional self-regulation.

## Devaluation of the generalist

Since 1945, general practice in all these countries has faced a problem of status among the health professions and within

21

higher education. For reasons which are partly historical and partly due to the successes associated with specialization in medical science and practice, the role of the generalist has been devalued in developed countries. This has affected the quantity and the quality of recruitment into this branch. Whereas this problem has to a large extent receded in the UK and the Netherlands since 1975, it persists in other countries, notably in France, Germany and the USA. In Finland and Sweden it persists despite fundamental reversals of government policy and the systematic redevelopment of primary care. This sort of difficulty, involving both attitude change and the relinquishing of vested interests, is not resolved quickly.

## Competition

Competition between GPs has not been an important feature in the UK in the last 50 years; it was more prevalent from 1900 to 1945. In Belgium, France, Italy and Germany it is intense because of the large number of doctors who qualify. In the USA, competition is a deep-rooted principle in society and in all areas of working life.

## Other causes of stress

Besides competition, other causes of stress in the UK, for example, more night calls or increased paper work are familiar to doctors in other European countries, particularly those in cities. Difficulty in admitting patients to hospitals is greater in the UK.

## Shared challenges summarized

The basic challenge of responding as effectively and sensitively as possible to the needs of patients, expressed or recognized, is at present complicated by a number of other challenges. To a varying extent the same ones come together in all developed countries. Among these the most important, now affecting primary as well as secondary care, is governmental intervention to control costs.

## International trends in response

Economic restriction and the search for value for money are challenges to primary care in every developed country. It is difficult to detect any one common or truly international trend in response to these challenges. However, one major effort to achieve a worldwide trend has been set off by the Alma Ata Declaration[14] and the programmes which have followed it under the title *Health for all 2000*. This has undoubtedly raised the profile of primary care, even in developed countries[15]. It has promoted the principle that secondary (and tertiary) care should support primary care, instead of dominating or controlling it. It has especially emphasized prevention, health promotion and the importance to health of other major elements in societies and governments, for example, education or housing.

This WHO initiative has struck a chord in countries already concerned about the costs and fragmentation associated with specialized curative medicine. Common sense suggests that, since secondary hospital care is inevitably expensive, transfer to primary care, home care or even to specialist day care, must save money. Systematic studies confirm this view overall, although the difference in costs in not always great[16,17]. Common sense also suggests that prevention and health promotion will reduce the incidence or severity of illness and so save money previously spent on care (this is still subject to debate)[18].

### Variations in response

The WHO campaign has raised the profile of primary care, but it has not been so strong as to create uniform responses in the countries being considered. Any statement about the similarities and differences between national responses to shared challenges is bound to be elaborate, requiring consideration not only of individual countries, but also of different issues.

The issues which need to be considered for the impact on primary care organization are:

- gate-keeping

- registration of patients

- control of distribution of doctors

- methods of paying doctors

- delay in specialist referral

- 24-hour coverage of population.

In each of these respects the countries in question vary. However, two groups of countries can be distinguished, because on the issues listed the countries in each group vary in the same direction. If the countries were placed in rank order on any one of these issues, the same countries, with few exceptions, would be found within the upper half of the range and the same ones would fall into the lower half.

It was proposed earlier in this chapter that universal access to a general doctor, with access to specialists only or mainly through referral, has been a particularly important and distinct feature of the NHS in the UK (ie gate-keeping). This feature has allowed the role of medical generalist to be developed and valued to an extent seldom seen in other countries.

Gate-keeping, by its presence or absence, distinguishes the two groups of countries. Where it is present, it is associated with certain other features; where it is absent, these too are absent.

In Table 2.1, western European countries are ranked by the proportion of all the specialist branches of medicine to which patients have direct access. The lowest figures show the countries in which gate-keeping is most complete. There is an obvious gap between Austria (0.62) and Denmark (0.29). This

**Table 2.1**   Accessibility of health care systems: specialist care (proportion of directly accessible professions)[1]

| Rank order | Health care system | Rate |
|------------|--------------------|------|
| 1 | Germany | 0.82 |
| 2 | Ireland (medium/high income) | 0.81 |
| 3 | Belgium | 0.79 |
| 4 | Switzerland | 0.78 |
|   | Finland (private) | 0.78 |
| 6 | Sweden | 0.74 |
| 7 | Denmark (Copenhagen) | 0.68 |
| 8 | France | 0.65 |
| 9 | Austria | 0.62 |
| 10 | Denmark (outside Copenhagen) | 0.29 |
| 11 | Portugal | 0.18 |
| 12 | Italy | 0.15 |
| 13 | The Netherlands (private) | 0.13 |
| 16 | Ireland (low income) | 0.09 |
|   | The Netherlands (public) | 0.09 |
|   | Norway | 0.09 |
|   | Spain | 0.09 |
| 18 | Finland (public) | 0.03 |
| 19 | UK | 0.00 |

[1]The total number of relevant specialties in each of these countries varies between 31 and 34.

Source: Royal College of General Practitioners (RCGP) *Occasional Paper* **48**, Tables 4.4, 5.5[19].

gap separates countries in the lower half of the list, in all of which gate-keeping is a prominent feature, from those in the upper half, where it is not. (The private practice elements in Ireland, Finland and the Netherlands are neglected, since they concern minorities is each of these three populations.)

Thus, western European countries fall into two groups over the question of gate-keeping. However, other features also distinguish the same groups. Wherever there is gate-keeping, there is control of the geographical distribution of GPs and, almost always, registration of patients. The two groups are also distinguished by their predominant methods of paying GPs. Countries in which there is gate-keeping, registration and control of distribution of doctors use capitation or salary, predominantly or entirely. The other group (excepting Sweden) uses payment by item of service.

Another correlation is with the length of delay between referral and specialist appointments. Almost without exception the delay is significantly longer in gate-keeping countries, usually more than twice as long. Direct access in the other countries mainly accounts for the difference.

Twenty-four hour coverage is an essential element in gate-keeping. When this is a legal or contractual obligation, it depends on the registration of patients with a doctor, a group practice or a health centre. This is the same in all the gate-keeping countries (often, however, delegated to a rota of colleagues or a deputizing service). In most of the other countries it exists as an ethical obligation only.

These contrasts between two groups of European countries are detailed in the Appendix (*see* page 35). They cannot be extended to many other issues; there are too many exceptions or variations. For example, although single-handed practice is rare and partnerships and groups of doctors are generally larger in gate-keeping countries, there are important exceptions (Italy, Ireland and Spain). Again, it would be difficult to show that multi-professional teams were significantly more common in gate-keeping countries, because of varying definitions of team membership.

Caution is again necessary in extending these grouped correlations outside Europe. They cannot, for example, be applied in Far East countries such as Japan, Hong Kong or Singapore. Most of the correlations in Canada, Australia and New Zealand put those countries into the gate-keeping group, but gate-keeping is incomplete and there are other anomalies.

Within the USA, the distinction is clearly demonstrated between the absence of gate-keeping in private practice and its presence in health maintenance organizations. It is here that the importance of this distinction becomes clear. Single-specialty, fee-for-service practitioners have a 40% excess of hospital admissions, with associated excess costs, over generalists working as gate-keepers in health maintenance organizations. (This difference takes into account the fact that health maintenance organizations deal with the fitter members of the population[20,21].) The hypothesis that gate-keeping by generalist doctors working in primary care is related to lower total health service costs was proposed by Maxwell in 1978[22] and put forward again by Starfield in 1992[23] and by Fry and Horder in 1994[24]. Schroeder[25] included patient self-referral to specialists, fee-for-service payments and high dependence on specialists for primary care among six conditions associated with high service costs.

Even if the experimental introduction of gate-keeping in countries (other than the USA) where it does not exist at present were to confirm that the relation with lower cost is one of cause and effect, other influences might be contributing to the same result. Examples might be the presence of global budgeting in hospitals or the proportion of public financing to total health expenditure[26].

The relationship between these differences among groups of countries and the wide variations in total health service costs (see page 34, Appendix) is only one of the basic considerations. Their possible relationship to the satisfaction of users is equally important and to indicators of health status equally or more important. The difficulty of establishing these relationships is discussed later in this chapter.

## Questions for the future

A small number of organizational developments introduced into the UK from abroad and now firmly rooted were mentioned briefly at the beginning of this chapter. Possible future developments which might stem from developments in other countries are discussed below.

## Freedom to choose

The trend towards limiting access to specialists in hospital care through referral is not seen in Belgium, France or Germany. Patients in those countries value their freedom to choose what sort of doctor they consult. Any effort to limit that freedom is likely to be resented and resisted by patients and by those specialists who work outside hospitals in the setting proper to primary care. Economic pressure may yet compel change there too. The change in the USA towards health maintenance organizations is now spreading rapidly. The decisions in Finland and Sweden to rebuild family care and to train GPs were clear reversals of previous policies favouring nearly total specialization. Starting in the 1970s, these trends are now requiring and introducing the registration of patients, in order to narrow the gateway to specialist care.

On the other hand, it is possible that people in our own country, given increasing information through the media and an increasing desire to participate in decisions affecting their lives, will cease to accept and support the present system which gives so strong a position to the GP as first access in the care of most medical or medically related problems. Could such a trend be prevented by further development of shared care between practitioners in primary and secondary services and by a greater use of second opinions?

## Personal care versus teamwork

Compared with Belgium, France, Germany or Italy, both group practice and teamwork with other professionals are much more prominent features of primary care in the UK. It is tempting to see the contrast as backwardness by those other countries in joining an inevitable trend. However, concern is already being expressed in the UK about the possible loss of personal care and continuity through the division in responsibility which can and does develop in large teams (the collusion of anonymity)[27-29]. We may see a counter-trend in this country, perhaps by those who can afford to pay for greater personal continuity and longer, less hurried consultations.

## The nurse-practitioner

Nurse-practitioners in Canada and the USA have a good reputation and an obvious role, since the distribution of primary care doctors is uneven. Moreover, the quality of their work has been compared with that of doctors in well conducted studies and found to compare well[30,31]. They are at present less expensive to employ than doctors.

Hitherto there has been no shortage of GPs to cover the UK. Even distribution has been one of the major achievements of the NHS. At first sight there is no need for nurse-practitioners, at least on the USA or Canadian pattern. However, they are now being trained in the UK in small numbers and they are enthusiastic to share the tasks of caring.

Time now spent by GPs on care management, as well as the continuing expansion of clinical tasks and the intention of the government to save money by transferring as much care as is safe from secondary to primary services, all contribute to the influences compelling GPs to share, delegate and increase teamwork. However, these processes, if done properly, take time. This can only be taken from consultation time or from the doctor's family.

The possible future role of nurse-practitioners is attractive to many members of the nursing profession as it promises to fulfil rising aspirations and to offer a more interesting career to those who are now getting a different sort of basic training. The role is liable to be interpreted by doctors as a threat, especially if it is suggested that in future nurses will increasingly take over the caring, pastoral function, calling on GPs only when necessary for technical tasks. This would, of course, change the traditional balance between the interpersonal and the technical elements in general practice, about which patients in many countries already complain.

However, shortage of time is not a new experience for GPs in the UK. It has been a constant cause of complaint from both patients and doctors, despite an increase in average consult-ation time from 5 minutes to 8 or 9 minutes, because responsi-bilities have increased in parallel. In this respect, the UK has always compared badly with Canada, France, Germany, the Netherlands, Sweden and the USA (*see* page 35, Appendix). Nurse-practitioners might provide an answer to this problem, not as a substitute for GPs but in addition to them. The division of labour is best decided in the place of work rather than in the councils of professional representative organizations.

## The outward flow of ideas

Some of this chapter has been concerned with developments which owe their origin to countries outside the UK. Even if one makes allowance for the tendency common in all countries to think that their own way of doing things is the best way, there are some good reasons for thinking that primary care in the UK is interesting to other countries. Registration of the whole population with GPs in 1948 was probably unique. The UK was among the first to develop a national programme of vocational training for general practice, based on a definition of the role, which influenced other European countries[32]. An outstanding output of research, journals and books is represented inter-nationally by the fact that the *British Journal of General Practice* is more often quoted in bibliographies than any other journal specific to this field of medicine[33]. Reference has already been made to the change in first career choice of young doctors in the UK between 1965 and 1990 with its sustained and marked swing towards primary care, not experienced elsewhere[34].

Finally, the present cluster of experiments in organization designed mainly to control rising costs in the UK is inevitably being watched by other governments, most of which have more reason to be concerned because they spend more of their national product on health. Among these experiments, the new role of GPs as purchasers, whether in fundholding practices or in larger groups, may prove to be of particular interest. It is now being tried in Finland and New Zealand and planned in parts of Australia[35]. Those countries share the objective of giving GPs a major role in shaping primary, secondary and community health care and countering the perceived dominance of specialists in service development.

## International comparisons of quality

At present every developed country is showing renewed interest in primary care, whether because it is seen as an important key to the control of rising costs or because its neglect is creating discontent in those who use health services.

If the hypothesis is confirmed that strong primary care with gate-keeping is related to control of costs as cause and effect, the strengthening of primary care seems likely to become a trend in every developed country as long as economic pressure dominates.

However, raising the quality of health services is a more fundamental purpose than controlling costs. Is there then any international convergence of ideas about how to raise quality? How much evidence is there that one form of organization is better than another, whatever the country? Does this fundamental purpose also point to the need to strengthen primary care in order to raise the quality of the service as a whole? Is there evidence that access through generalist doctors acting as gate-keepers secures a higher quality service overall than direct access by patients to specialists? Common sense might even suggest the opposite.

In this chapter, the answer to these important, but difficult, questions must be both brief and disappointing. Comparisons of quality in health services depend ideally on measurements of the outcomes of care, particularly measurement and comparison of health status and the assessment of satisfaction in those who use the service. Between countries, comparisons of the state of health still rely on such broad and crude indicators as expectation of life or infant mortality, because for these clearly defined features national statistics are reliable; like can be compared with like. The possibility of finding outcome indicators sufficiently relevant and specific for use in comparing the effectiveness of different patterns of care across national boundaries remains for the future. Even if this is achieved (as seems possible) and differences in more specific measurements of health are found between countries, there is still the problem of attributing differences to particular national features in the structure and process of care. There are many other variables which might account for the differences in outcome.

It is reasonable, nevertheless, to put forward hypotheses for testing, on the basis of observations, comparisons and correlations, such as those which have been described above. This has been attempted internationally by Schroeder[25], Starfield[23] and Fry and Horder[24]. The hypotheses common to these three sources are that a national health system is likely to achieve higher quality and lower total costs if it contains or develops strong primary care. Strong primary care requires the following.

- A government programme which places a high value on primary care by paying for it and which ensures appropriate distribution of services and an appropriate balance between primary and secondary services.

- Payment of primary care doctors mainly by capitation or salary, with financial incentives for particular priorities (eg preventive activities or team development).

- 24-hour accountability for defined populations.

- Payment of specialists by salary rather than fee for service, to achieve a more appropriate and less costly allocation of resources.

- Restricted access of patients to specialists to encourage first contact by primary care providers (preferably generalist-trained) and to foster co-ordination.

- Organization of primary care in health centres rather than individual offices, with better use of nurse and other team members, to increase comprehensiveness.

The problems of method in assessing quality must first be attacked within individual countries. In the UK, the organizational developments described in this book can expect to have to pass an increasingly rigorous quality test as the primary care focus continues to expand.

## Appendix

Appendix follows on next three pages.

*Appendix*

| | Proportion of directly accessible professions[1] | GP register of patients[2] | Control of distribution of GPs[3] | Type of GP remuneration[4] | Delay in referral from GP to specialist[5] | 24-hour responsibility[6] | Mean length GP consultation (min)[7] | GDP at market prices (1995) (£cash)[8] | Total health expenditure per person (1995)[9] | % GDP on health (1995)[10] |
|---|---|---|---|---|---|---|---|---|---|---|
| Germany | 0.82 | - | - | F | 6.9 | - | 9 | 19.717 | 1677 | 8.5 |
| Ireland (high income)[11] | 0.81 | | | | | | | | | |
| Belgium | 0.79 | - | - | F | 7.5 | - | 11 | 14.945 | 1.214 | 8.1 |
| Switzerland | 0.78 | - | - | F | 12.5 | - | 12.5 | 23.877 | 2.176 | 9.1 |
| Finland (private)[11] | 0.78 | | | | | | | | | |
| Sweden | 0.74 | (-) + | + | C | | + | 15+ | 16.069 | 1.317 | 8.2 |
| Denmark (Copenhagen)[12] | 0.68 | | | | | | | | | |
| France | 0.65 | - | - | F | 6.3 | - | 14 | 15.631 | 1.435 | 9.2 |
| Austria | 0.62 | - | -? | F | | | | 17.192 | 1.513 | 8.8 |
| Denmark (outside Copenhagen) | 0.29 | + | + | C | 26.2 | + | 6.4 | 19.594 | 1.249 | 6.4 |
| Portugal | 0.18 | + | + | C | 28.5 | + | 8.2 | 5.854 | 337 | 5.8 |
| Italy | 0.15 | + | + | C | 10.7 | - | 7.6 | 13.230 | 1.122 | 8.5 |
| Netherlands (private)[11] | 0.13 | | | | | | | | | |

*continued*

*Appendix continued*

| | Proportion of directly accessible professions[1] | GP register of patients[2] | Control of distribution of GPs[3] | Type of GP remuneration[4] | Delay in referral from GP to specialist[5] | 24-hour responsibility[6] | Mean length GP consultation (min)[7] | GDP at market prices (1995) (£cash)[8] | Total health expenditure per person (1995)[9] | % GDP on health (1995)[10] |
|---|---|---|---|---|---|---|---|---|---|---|
| Ireland (low income) | 0.09 | + | + | C | 27.4 | + | 8 | 9.695 | 659 | 6.8 |
| Netherlands (public) | 0.09 | + | + | C | 10.8 | + | 8 | 14.699 | 1.234 | 8.4 |
| Norway | 0.09 | (-)+ | + | C & F | 33.7 | + | 15 | 17.550 | 1.367 | 7.8 |
| Spain | 0.09 | + | + | C | 12 | + | 4.7 | 9.541 | 643 | 6.7 |
| Finland (public) | 0.03 | +(-) | + | C | | + | 15+ | 12.080 | 1.001 | 8.3 |
| UK | 0.00 | + | + | C | 36.3 | + | 8.6 | 12.103 | 814 | 6.8 |
| Canada | Low | - | +- | F | ? | | 12 | 14.626 | 1.447 | 9.9 |
| USA (private) | High | - | - | F | ? | | 13+ | 17.957 | 2.816 | 15.7 |
| USA (HMO) | Low | | - | C & F | ? | | 13+ | | | |
| Australia | Low | - | - | F | ? | | ? | 11.555 | 949 | 8.2 |
| New Zealand | Low | - | - | F | ? | | ? | 9.061 | 659 | 7.3 |
| Japan | High | - | - | F | ? | - | ? | 23.964 | 1.650 | 6.9 |
| Singapore | Low | - | - | F | ? | | ? | | | |

[1]Royal College of General Practitioners (1992) The Interface Study. Occasional Paper **48**: 41.

[2]Presence or absence in general practices of a registered list of patients. Boerma G W, de Jong F A J M and Mulder P (1993) Health Care and General Practice across Europe. Utrecht. NIVEL.

*continued*

*Appendix continued*

[3]Presence or absence of national or regional control of distribution of general practitioners. Royal College of General Practitioners (1992) (see above).

[4]Predominant method of paying general practitioners:F, fee-for-service;C, either capitation or salary (or both). Groenewegen P P, van der Zee J and van Haeften R (1991) Remunerating general practitioners in western Europe. Aldershot, Avebury and Boerma *et al.* (1993) (see above).

[5]Delay (days) in achieving referral to a specialist. Royal College of General Practitioners (1992) The European study of referrals from primary to secondary care. Occasional Paper **56**: 66.

[6]Legal or contractual responsibility for 24-hour coverage of patients by GPs. Groenewegen *et al.* (1991) (see above); Boerma *et al.* (1993). (see above).

[7]Various sources, including Gervas J *et al.* (1994) Primary care, financing and gatekeeping in western Europe. *Family Practice.* **11**: 307–17.

[8]Gross domestic product at market prices (£ sterling) in 1995. Office of Health Economics (1995) Compendium of health statistics. Office of Health Economics, London.

[9]Percentage of gross domestic product devoted to health. Office of Health Economics (see above).

[10]Total health expenditure per person. Office of Health Economics (see above).

[11]Further comparisons were not sought for Ireland (high income), Finland (private) or Netherlands (private) because these are minorities in each country.

[12]In Denmark, Copenhagen has now ceased to have an organization which differs from the rest of the country.

# Acknowledgements

I am grateful for helpful comments to Professor van den Bussche (Hamburg), Professor van Es (Amersfoort), Professor Gordon Moore (Boston), Mr Geoffrey Meads (NHS Executive) and to my wife, Dr Elizabeth Horder.

# References

1   World Health Organization (1962) The role of public health officers and general practitioners in mental health care. *WHO Tech Rep Ser.* **235**, Geneva.

2   World Health Organization (1964) General practice: Report of an expert committee. *WHO Tech Rep Ser.* **267**, Geneva.

3   Horder J P (1965) The general practitioner in Yugoslavia, Czechoslovakia and Israel, special vocational training. *Lancet.* **2**: 123–5.

4   Kark S L (1989) *The practice of community-oriented primary health care.* Appleton-Century, New York.

5   Cherkasky M (1952) *The family health maintenance demonstration. Research in public health.* Millbank Memorial Foundation, New York.

6   Silver G A (1958) Beyond general practice – the health team. *Yale J Biol Med.* **31**: 29.

7   Donabedian A (1966) Evaluating the quality of medical care. *Millbank Memorial Fund Quarterly,* **44**: 166–203.

8   Enthoven A C (1985) *Reflections on the management of the national health service.* Nuffield Provincial Hospitals Trust, London.

9   Roehmer M (1994) *National health systems of the world. Volume I* Oxford University Press, New York. p 131.

10  Morley D, Rohde J and Williams G (1985) *Practising health for all.* Oxford University Press, Oxford.

11  Cunningham N (1969) An evaluation of an auxiliary based child health service in rural Nigeria. *J Soc Health Nigeria.* **3**: 21–5.

12  The Economist (1993) *Pocket world in figures.* The Economist, London.

13  Office of Health Economics (1995) *Compendium of health statistics.* Office of Health Economics, London.

14  World Health Organization (1978) *Primary health care.* WHO, Geneva.

15  Godlee F (1995) WHO in Europe; does it have a role? *BMJ.* **310**: 389–93.

16  Berk A A and Chalmers T C (1981) Cost and efficiency of the substitution of ambulatory for in-patient care. *New England J Med.* **304**: 393–7.

17  Horder J P (1988) Cost-effectiveness of hospital versus community care. In: Binns T B and Firth M (eds) *Provision under financial constraint: need, demand and resources.* Royal Society of Medicine, London.

18  Hoffenberg R, Smith A and Shapiro S (1988) Can prevention be cost effective? Contributions to Anglo-American conference. In: Binns T B and Firth M *Provision under financial constraint: need, demand and resources.* Royal Society of Medicine, London.

19   Fleming D (1992) The European study of referrals from primary to secondary care. Royal College of General Practitioners. Occasional Paper. 48.

20   Manning W G, Leibowitz A, Goldberg G A, Rogers W H and Newhouse J P (1984) A controlled trial of the effect of a pre-paid group practice on use of services. *New England J Med.* **310**: 1505–10.

21   Greenfield S, Nelson E C, Zubkoff M, *et al.* (1992) Variations in resource utilisation among medical specialties and systems of care. Results from the medical outcomes study. *J Am Med Assoc.* **267**: 264–30.

22   Maxwell R J (1978) *Health and wealth.* Lexington.

23   Starfield B (1992) Primary care, concept, evaluation and policy. Oxford University Press, New York.

24   Fry J and Horder J P (1994) Primary health care in an international context. Nuffield Provincial Hospitals Trust, London.

25   Schroeder S A (1984) Western European responses to physician oversupply, lessons for the United States. *Journal Am Assoc.* **252**: 373–84.

26   Gerdtham U G, Sugaard J, Johnsson O N B and Anderssen F (1990) A pooled cross-sectional analysis of the health care expenditure of OECD countries. Paper prepared for the 2nd World Congress on Health Economics, Zurich.

27   Symposium in the *J Inter-professional Care.* In press. 1995.

28   Pratt J (1995) *Practitioners and practices. A conflict of values?* Radcliffe Medical Press, Oxford.

29   Balint M (1964) *The doctor, his patient and the illness.* 2nd edn. Pitman Medical, London.

30  Spitzer W O, Sackett D I, Sibley J C, *et al* (1974) The Burlington randomised trial of the nurse practitioner. *New England J Med.* **290**: 251–6.

31  Spurgeon D (1995) Expanded role planned for Ontario's nurses. *BMJ.* **310**: 80.

32  Leeuwenhorst Working Party (1977) The work of the general practitioner. Statement by a Working Party of the 2nd European Conference on the teaching of general practice. *J Roy Coll General Practitioners.* **27**: 117.

33  Royal Netherlands Academy of Arts and Sciences (1994) General practice research in Dutch academia. Proceedings of a workshop. Amsterdam.

34  Ellin D J, Parkhouse H F and Parkhouse J (1986) Career preferences of doctors qualifying in the United Kingdom in 1983. *Health Trends.* **18**: 59–63.

35  Mason A and Morgan K (1995) Purchaser-provider: The international dimension. *BMJ.* **310**: 231–5.

# The managed practice  3

*John Hughes*

The NHS reforms, which were introduced in 1990, represent the greatest organizational and philosophical change in British health care since 1948. The upheaval and uncertainty of the last five years is set to continue for some time as the administered service of the 1980s is transformed into a managed organization incorporating strategic planning and business methods more fitting for the approach of the twenty-first century. The challenge for the medical profession is how best to maximize its influence within this new corporate structure while maintaining the traditional role of advocacy for the individual patient. General practice has the additional problem of reconciling the new management style with its independent contractor status.

## The changes

The major health service changes in the UK that, in my view, will have an impact on general practice from 1996 are discussed below.

## Amalgamated DHAs and FHSAs

In many parts of the country this process has already begun, but the granting of formal statutory recognition to the new combined authorities or Health Commissions is due to commence in April 1996. The coalescence of secondary and primary care management under the same organizational umbrella should, at least theoretically, assist in the efficient provision of total patient care. Whether the new authorities will have sufficient expertize in matters relating to general practice, however, remains to be seen, as some FHSAs are evidently becoming subsumed by their DHA counterparts.

## Establishment of regional offices

Also in April 1996 the recently amalgamated Regional Health Authorities (RHAs) will change in status and function to become outposts of the NHS Executive. Gone will be the hierarchical structure of health service management and in its place will be a civil service office the function of which will be to ensure that the prevailing philosophy of the Department of Health is enacted at District level. The new Commissions will thus assume a powerful role in delivering total health care to the population under their charge, guided by doctrinal edicts from above, yet unconstrained by the layers of bureaucracy to which they are at present answerable.

## A primary care led service

The relevance of the organizational changes in the NHS to general practice becomes vividly apparent when viewed in the light of the Government's desire to see a shift in direction from, what is perceived to be, a hospital-dominated focus to a community or primary care oriented service. To what extent this desire is driven by altruism or financial considerations is, of course, arguable, but nevertheless the consequences for general practice are unavoidable. In forthcoming years a greater degree of health care is likely to remain within the primary care sector and that which does transfer into a hospital setting is likely to be returned to the community as quickly as possible. Although these changes are already apparent, the new arrangements will lead to an acceleration of this process, as strategic planning begins to embody the principle of a primary care led service. The success of GPs in influencing this new scenario and their ability to adapt to it are fundamental to the future of the profession itself.

## GPs in a managed service

The NHS Executive's EL(94)79 published in October 1994 states 'new health authorities . . . will have overall responsibility for assessing the health needs of the local population and for developing integrated strategies for meeting those needs across primary and secondary care boundaries. Managing the new NHS envisages a key role for the new health authorities in developing primary care and forging a constructive partnership with GPs'[1].

What place, then, do GPs and general practice have in the 'new NHS'? What relationships can be forged with the new authorities which will deliver a primary care led service? There will necessarily be tensions in many districts as these authorities or Health Commissions flex their muscles. The independence and reactive nature of GPs will not fit comfortably with the sense of 'being managed'. It is essential that these, potentially destructive, conflicts be explored early on and resolved satisfactorily so that primary care can indeed develop and flourish, lifting the morale of GPs as it does so.

In order to consider the development of general practices in forthcoming years four major issues must be addressed:

- independence versus a salaried service
- local versus national contracts
- narrow or broad core services
- whether the contract will be with the practice or the practitioner.

## Independence versus salaried service

Many managers in the health service, particularly those from a DHA background, have some difficulty in understanding the independent contractor status of GPs. They expect to 'manage' general practice as they once managed hospital departments. There are an increasing number of GPs who would opt to be salaried should this choice be available. The profession as a whole, and indeed health service managers and politicians, would be wise to resist this temptation. It is the feeling of independence and the responsibility for our own practice development, coupled often with considerable business expertize that has enabled the evolution of a high standard of primary medical care in the UK despite the pressure of rising patient expectations and the imposition of unreasonable contractual obligations. To remove this independent status would be to destroy the soul of general practice and indeed lead to an exodus from the NHS of some of our best doctors. This does not mean that there is no room within the profession for salaried practitioners. There is clearly a place for doctors willing to assume this status, but it should be reserved for particular circumstances and not regarded as the norm. The relationship between Health Commissions and general practice cannot, therefore, be regarded as a form of line management, but must be a contractual arrangement on a proper business footing, with common aims, agreed quality standards and underpinned by adequate resources. The independence of the profession must be respected and safeguarded and only on that basis can we proceed.

## Local versus national contracts

The national GMS contract has long been valued by GPs as a mechanism for providing a certain degree of uniformity, equality and mutual protection, despite the widespread criticism of the 1990 version and the inability of the profession to resist government imposition. Efforts to modify the 1990 contract meaningfully have met with little success, but despite this there has been considerable reluctance to regard local contracts as a viable alternative. It is also unlikely that the government would wish, in the short term at least, to see a wholesale move to local contracting, which may risk the loss of central control over the profession. In contrast to this, Health Commission executives may see local contracts as the best means of delivering locally responsive health care. Indeed it is difficult to see any real advantage to the formation of integrated primary and secondary care authorities without affording them the ability to enter into discussions with primary care professionals at local district level. Accepting that a national contract, in some form, will remain in place for the time being, local contracts may be developed to encompass new services or provide extra resources.

### New services
Local contracts may be developed to provide new services not traditionally undertaken in primary care. Arrangements of this sort are already in evidence in some districts. A move from hospital-based service provision into primary care, utilizing the considerable expertize which exists in general practice, has the advantage of bringing treatment closer to the patient, enlarging the knowledge base of general practice, and often, providing a more cost-effective service. Quality of care must be maintained and contracts which match quality indicators with resource investment are essential.

### Extra resources
Local contracts may be adapted to provide extra resources to support identified work-load shifts. Over the years there has

been a steady drip-feed of work into primary care. The momentum behind such changes will begin to increase as the new health authorities plan specifically for reductions in hospital patient contacts, namely:

- out-patient attendances will be reduced

- moves to day-case surgery will increase

- shorter in-patient stays will be expected

- care in the community for the elderly will continue.

For the first time Health Commissions will be in a position to manage this transfer of responsibility and work-load effectively. Efforts must be made, in partnership with GPs, to quantify the impact of these changes on primary care and to resource the resulting work-load adequately. Contractual arrangements must be put in place to underpin this process.

### Modifications of national contract at local level
Huge variations exist in the health needs of differing populations. Inner-city deprived communities differ in their use of health and social services from those in middle-class suburbia. To allow for modifications to the national contract to take into consideration these and other factors would seem to be logical. To penalize financially those doctors working with poorly compliant patients because of failures to reach immunization and cervical screening targets, for example, is ludicrous and cannot be excused by the payment of arbitrarily calculated deprivation payments. Such a scheme cannot foster well-planned and responsive primary care provision. Health promotion measures might similarly be modified in response to local requirements.

A rigid national contract is incompatible with locally managed, integrated health care and local modifications and variations, if properly negotiated, can have advantages for both GPs and managers.

## Narrow or broad core services

An integral part of any contractual discussion is the definition of the core services a GP is expected to provide or be responsible for providing. At the 1994 LMC conference the General Medical Services Committee (GMSC) was instructed to institute a debate on the subject and it subsequently produced an excellent discussion paper defining core general medical services[2]. The inexorable rise in workload for GPs over the past few years tempts one to define this core as narrowly as possible, including within the definition only patient-initiated consultations and maternity care. These would be separately remunerated (as at present) with restriction of provision being possible if levels of resourcing are inadequate and, more importantly would be dealt with outside of average net remuneration. However, there is a danger to this approach. It must be recognized that any services left out of the core would be open to competition from other providers. This alternative provision may come from other GPs, other organizations (eg family planning clinics), or other professionals (eg midwives). When considered alongside a move to locally managed services it is not difficult to envisage the development of a tendering process in which GPs are only one of many possible providers. If target net remuneration is reduced to a lower level than at present, encompassing only patient-initiated consultations (whatever that might be priced at) many practitioners may find difficulty in regaining their present income in the face of an increasingly competitive world of primary care provision.

Breaking what is regarded by some as a GP monopoly over the provision of primary care is high in the minds of some in the NHS and GPs will be well advised not to be complacent about this nor take decisions which may weaken the professions' position in later years. General practice is, by and large, of a very high standard in the UK and one of its strengths is the philosophy of 'holism' which it embodies. When we are considering what GPs should regard as their core responsibilities it may be as well to reflect this concept in the definition.

## Practice or practitioner

Practice-based contracts as an alternative to individual contracts have become one of several matters for discussion following the GMSC paper *Which Way Forward* which was published in 1993[3]. Although GPs have an individual 'contractual' relationship with the NHS for the provision of care to individual patients, in effect most doctors exercise the provision of services on a practice basis. In the event of locally determined contractual arrangements there may develop a mixture of individual and practice-based contracts. A partner with a specific skill (eg endoscopy) may have an individual contract with a Health Commission but the provision of specific health promotion measures or extended chronic disease management might more sensibly be contracted on a practice basis. Practice-based contracts legitimize delegation within a practice to nurses and other staff whose skills may be more appropriately employed than those of the doctors themselves.

# The evolving practice

General practice has come a long way in the last 30 years. Vocational training has improved standards and attracted a high calibre of doctor into the profession. Shared investment in staff and premises has allowed many practices to expand and extend the range of services they are able to offer. Continuing education has allowed GPs to become the present day general physicians, as our consultant colleagues have become super-specialists. Despite all these advances, however, GPs and their practices continue to function as small units with no cross-fertilization of ideas, no collective goals and no uniform strategy for the future. In the emerging 'reformed' NHS these attitudes will become more and more difficult to sustain. We will be expected to become more responsible for the 'public health' as well as the health of individuals, and we will be expected to take part in collaborative strategic planning with colleagues and managers. Indeed, it may be that future investment in our practices will be dependent upon our willingness and ability to do so.

A scenario therefore unfolds in which local contracting, in addition to or as a modification of a national contract, emerges as a means of delivering Health Commission aims. Local contracts, must by their nature, be collaborative with input from all interested parties. GPs who wish to become involved with such arrangements may find opportunities for imaginative and innovative practice developments which are at present impossible. Proper contractual agreements are likely to be bound by quality indicators and in order to discharge their responsibilities effectively practices will require sound management and information systems. It will be necessary to address issues of appropriate skill mix within the practice as broader responsibilities necessitate greater delegation. The developing primary care team must be managed competently either by or on behalf of the GPs who themselves must remain at the fulcrum of primary care provision. At this point there comes a major challenge for GPs which revolves around the relationship between the practice, consisting of GPs and ancillary staff, and the extended primary care team and attached professionals. The options are to maintain the relationship which exists at present, for the most part, whereby community staff are employed and managed by community managers and work in various degrees of co-operation with the practice, or to change this relationship by transferring the management of community staff into the practice itself. Whether the second option is chosen or not will depend on the willingness of community staff to become part of the practice team and the willingness of politicians to allow this to happen. There is no doubt that the present political direction is towards devolving more and more purchasing power and responsibility for service provision into general practices and away from Commissions. The latter, should the present course be held, will find their present purchasing position severely restricted, but they will continue to be involved in budget setting and ensuring that the wishes of the NHS Executive are carried out. They will also be expected to lead the strategy planning of health care in their Districts. In order to develop a more robust negotiating position some practices may well see the advantage of extending their management net into the community arena thereby creating a dynamic and powerful 'provider unit'. Initially this is likely to include the expertize of district nursing and health visiting as well as the established practice staff as it is the function of these groups with which GPs are most familiar. There is, however, no limit to the expansion of the team. Psychiatric nurses, midwives, counsellors and therapists may all be brought together, not in a loose alliance as at present, but as an integral part of the extended provider unit which acts as one to deliver managed primary and community care. This unit will be in a strong position to negotiate with Health Commissions, with the practice population as the base, facilitating the achievement of true integrated planning for the benefit of its patients. It is possible to extend this model further to encompass social care in addition to medical care. The boundary between the two is often arbitrary and unhelpful, especially in the case of elderly dependent patients. A more sensibly managed delivery system may well prevent some of the disasters which have occurred in recent years where patients have been bounced between two organizations without proper assessment, discussion or liaison. At present, Social Services Departments are both purchasers and providers of social care, in most instances with no financial involvement with the health sector. This follows from the government's decision to allocate previous Social Security monies for residential and nursing home care through Local Authorities rather than through health channels. To allow general practices to become more responsible for social care would go some way towards solving these problems. Primary care management would then be responsible for the totality of patient care with the ability to purchase or commission social provision from whichever provider was most appropriate. The responsibility for total care provision would then rest with one organization, based around general practice, thereby making seamless care a reality.

As the political sands shift and general practices develop at different speeds, a multitude of differing schemes of providing and purchasing are likely to be created. No one arrangement will necessarily be better than another, nor more successful, but to deny the profession the freedom to experiment and innovate will be to deny a 'primary care led service'.

The profession will always regard change as a threat if it is imposed from without, but to be in control of change is challenging and stimulating and we have the opportunity to do just that.

## References

1   National Health Service Executive (1994) EL (94) 79 *Developing NHS purchasing and GP fundholding.* NHSE, London.

2   GMSC Discussion Paper (1994) *Core general medical services and the classification of general practitioners activity.* GMSC, London.

3   GMSC Discussion Paper (1993) *General practice: which way forward?* GMSC, London.

# The total fundholder  |4

*David Colin-Thomé*

## Beginnings

The germination of the idea behind total fundholding came mainly from within the ranks of fundholding GPs, with varying degrees of involvement from both DHAs and FHSAs. This 'bottom up' approach has now been accepted as an exciting development in health care delivery, a prime example of how both the ideas and energies of the grass roots can be allowed to flourish in parts of the reformed NHS. The original fundholding initiative emanated from the Department of Health but its development heavily involved GPs and health service managers; a welcome change from the old monolithic 'top down' NHS. The total fundholding initiative has taken that emancipated process a step further.

The Secretary of State for Health, Mrs Virginia Bottomley, following on from the four initial projects in 1994/5, initially suggested 25 further national projects in October 1994. In fact, a further 51 projects are taking part in a preparatory year from 1995/6 with the agreement of the local health authority. The idea is that these projects will go live in 1996/7.

Total fundholding clearly seems to be an idea whose time has come. In only the fourth year of fundholding, it is a rapid development when set in the context of the sometimes unresponsive bureaucracy of yesteryear. In 1994, at two significant national fundholding conferences organized by the National Health Service Executive (NHSE) at the behest of the then Minister for Health, the majority of GPs present expressed an interest in total fundholding. Both the NHSE at regional level and local health authorities are now having to refuse some volunteers in order for the numbers to remain manageable, given the decision by the NHSE for the 51 projects to be formally evaluated.

At the two conferences mentioned above, many GPs also wished to explore the idea that GMS monies, (the monies from which all GPs receive their remuneration and payment of practice expenses), should also be part of some total fundholding projects. Only one of the four initial projects actually explored that line, within the constraining forces of the law.

## Benefits

What are the perceived benefits of total fundholding that seem to have captivated the imagination of many? Ian Carruthers, acting Regional Director of the South and West Regional Office of the NHSE in 1994/5, and Chief Executive of Dorset Health Commission, states that the benefits of expanded fundholding are substantial because the GP purchasers are able to[1]:

- take a holistic view of the community and its values, in identifying needs and setting priorities; (from experience this usually broadens the agenda to embrace wider health issues, but this is a challenge to be met if health status is to be improved; it represents a major challenge for purchasing at practice level)

- increase communication at operational and strategic levels between agencies (this is fundamental to creating effective alliances)

- develop a more coherent view of patient care as it obliterates the perceived artificial barrier between what is in and what is not in fundholding

- project a model of fundholding which makes more sense to non-fundholders who can see this a more useful goal to achieve

- become closer to all their consumers rather than just existing service users

- enable minority users to be better identified and represented

- eliminate duplication of effort and resources

- provide scope to innovate often by challenging the orthodox

- empower local people and organizations to make effective representation so that they can contribute to the future shaping of health

- encourage the exchange of information and audit of health service delivery from a variety of perspectives

- provide a resource for dealing with individual casework problems in local settings

- balance the individual versus population dilemma as access to intelligence of needs at both levels is forthcoming

- facilitate delivery of more individualized care for the consumer.

He goes on to say 'these benefits are being derived from fundholding and locality purchasing models. It should be noted that local purchasing is not an optional extra but at the heart of delivering the agenda of the modernized NHS by placing general practitioners in a more central role to influence health in their communities'.

Carruthers then identifies some success criteria for total fundholding.

- Changes in referral and treatment patterns, based on audited effective interventions with new patterns of service achieved as a result of practice-based purchasing.

- More and better quality care being achieved.

- Improved choice for patients, (eg they can trade off waiting time against travel distance).

- Improvement in the integration of primary, community and secondary care services.

- Shifts to primary care services through such new patterns of care as hospital-at-home.

- The drive to ensure efficient local provision of services (reducing duplication, optimizing location).

- Greater focus on purchasing for health improvements rather than concentration on health service delivery.

- GP involvement and support for the arrangements.

- Views, needs and wants of the consumer, Community Health Councils (CHCs), voluntary bodies and the wider public influencing the purchasing pattern.

- Providers responding to new needs as well as overall population requirements, with a major culture shift and swift flexible provider responses to local needs.

- Reduced overheads with more spent on delivering effective high-quality, value-for-money health care.

As set out, this is a daunting agenda, which if it is to be achieved needs to be counterbalanced by the following comments. Fundholding gave some credence and specific resources to the idea of the primary care organization being in the best position to deliver managed care. I deliberately use the phrase 'managed care' even though it is a concept developed in the USA, with the recognition that foreign ideas cannot easily be transferred. Managed care depends on good quality primary care which then finds ways, either through providing or purchasing, of ensuring high quality, cost-effective care for the patient. Fundholding began that process, but has had many critics, some of whose criticisms it seems are based on the inability to accept change. Others, however, are valid:

- budgets set do not reflect need because they were based on historic activity patterns

- fundholding is very costly, especially in its associated transaction and management costs

- there is an unclear role differentiation between the large Health Authority purchasers and fundholding which has led in some areas to unnecessary competition between these two organizations.

Total fundholding, especially in the context of the new NHS, as set out in the National Health Service Executive (NHSE) document EL(94)79 issued in October 1994, enables general practice population purchasing to be the preferred option for locality purchasing[2]. The idea of the practice population as a basis for health care planning and delivery also has added support from the NHSE publication on the future of nursing, *New world, new opportunities*, which suggests that practice populations are the appropriate local population on which to base primary care delivery[3].

The emphasis of the new Health Authority in these arrangements will not be on direct purchasing as this will now be the function of GPs in whatever form they decide to purchase. The role of Health Authorities will be strategy, monitoring and regulation, support and development. NHSE letter EL(94)79, concerned with developing NHS purchasing and GP fundholding towards a primary care led NHS, sets out a clear role for the new Health Authorities[2]. The new Authorities, from April 1996, will continue their leading role in the development and implementation of a local health strategy working in collaboration with GPs, NHS Trusts, local agencies and local people. As the single statutory Health Authority at local level they will be well placed to develop a coherent view of the health needs of the local population and of the distinct contribution the various parts of the NHS and local agencies can make to achieving those needs. In many parts of the country, Health Authorities and GPs, fundholding and non-fundholding, are already working closely to ensure they meet the needs both of individual patients and of the local community. This good practice will be developed to promote stronger partnerships across the country as a whole. Health Authorities will continue to assess health needs; deploy resources to meet those needs; build consensus on and implement local health strategies; develop partnerships with local agencies; and maintain quality and effectiveness. Government intends that Health Authorities will continue to have the overall responsibility for working with GPs to ensure that the health needs of the whole community are identified and met. They will have a major role in supporting these changes. They will also continue to have a direct purchasing role, for example, on behalf of non-fundholding GPs, for services excluded from the fundholding scheme or for specialist services which cover more than a single district, for some time to come.

Health Authorities will agree with GPs, local people and agencies what needs to be done to ensure that national and local priorities are met through GP-led purchasing. This requires the full involvement of GPs, NHS Trusts, local agencies and other interested parties. Health Authorities will issue budget allocations for GP fundholders and ensure that the way in which GPs fulfil their providing and purchasing roles is in the interest of patients and ensures value for money.

Authorities will support the development of primary care through advice, investment and training. They will assist all practices which wish to become fundholders. All practices will be involved in wider purchasing decisions.

Within this context, it is clear that total fundholding projects will actually be devolved health authorities for their patient population, utilizing the skills and managerial knowledge of the Health Authority to develop this process. Where non-total fundholding is taking place the Health Authority will have a more complex role but will essentially still be devolving much of the responsibility to the GP-led organization.

# Pioneers

Drawing on reports of the initial total fundholding projects, let us look at the models in more detail[4-7].

## Bromsgrove

This is one of the projects for which the budget was already live in 1994/5. This project therefore needs to be examined in most detail as it is the most advanced in its development. The project covers 39 000 patients living in Bromsgrove who are all registered with one of the four practices included in the project. Other patients registered with the practices but living outside the town are not included in this scheme. All four practices (a total of 22 GPs) are existing fundholding practices and each practice continues to manage fundholding separately. The project covers all remaining health and community care needs of the patients living in Bromsgrove. It is a 2-year project, which began on 1 April 1994 when the budget was received to purchase services based on a weighted capitation formula. The budget amounts to £13.92 million with management costs of £90 000, funded by the West Midlands regional office of the NHSE. There is no top-slicing of the budget although joint contracting with the DHA in some of the risk areas has been agreed, in particular in mental health.

The objectives of the project are to:

* provide the means to improve the integration of primary and secondary care

* ensure that secondary care purchasing is primary care led

- provide the framework which creates incentives to make changes in the patterns of care

- establish whether contracting on a true cost-per-case basis will result in more effective purchasing

- assess the management and administration requirements and the implications of delegating total responsibility for purchasing to GPs.

A Bromsgrove GP purchasing committee was established as a sub-committee of the North Worcestershire Health Authority and includes a representative from each practice, representatives from the Health Authority and Hereford and Worcester FHSA. This committee has the delegated legal responsibility for the management of the budget and is accountable for disbursement of the budget. A project team has been set up for agreeing the purchasing plan and monitoring contract performance against plan. A representative from each practice, from the Health Authority and FHSA, and the project manager form the project team. The project manager has been appointed to oversee the project, assisted by data entry clerks and information technology (IT) support. The project also employs a full-time liaison nurse and assistant who are responsible for working closely with patients and consultants to achieve early discharge from secondary care into the community.

The project computer is based at one surgery and data entry is made via land lines to the main processor from the other surgeries. The software to manage the project has been developed by a computer company working closely with the team.

The areas covered by the budget are hospital-related expenditure and community-related services. Hospital related expenditure includes accident and emergency services, ambulance services, extra-contractual referrals, utilization of local community hospital, emergency admissions, non-fundholding elective in-patient care and day surgery services, maternity care, dental care, regional specialties, plastic surgery and sexually transmitted diseases. Community related services include school nursing, family planning, health surveillance, immunization, audiology, school medicals, a community drugs team, child and adolescence psychiatry, home loan store, breast screening, home support services, day care, learning difficulties, long-stay patients and respite care.

Dr Wilkinson, a GP in the project, has stated that the local Acute Trust had difficulty in meeting the project's information needs and that data from the local NHS community trust had been patchy but was improving. There has been difficulty in providing practice level information for some services. Most contracts are cost per case, emergency admission costs are based by specialties on length of stay bands. Invoices are paid on behalf of the project by the DHA.

Any underspend achieved is used to improve the provision of services to patients in the Bromsgrove area. Bromsgrove project members are expecting initial underspends of at least £500 000 or over 5%. In the first six months of the project, the four practices kept emergency referrals 17% below the previous year. Emergency referrals which consume a quarter of NHS spending are rising elsewhere in the UK. The GP revisiting or using a good district nursing service can avoid some emergency referrals, in the view of Dr Wilkinson. The project is also keeping costs down by specifying different price bands for different lengths of stay, and by employing a project nurse to make sure that people are discharged as early as possible. This liaison nurse visits patients in the local Acute Trust and questions whether they could go home or transfer to less high-tech accommodation in the local community hospital or private nursing homes under their GP's care. The choice has been left to the patients, but the hospital consultants must also agree with the decision. As a result of this work, average hospital lengths of stay have been cut from 9 days to 4 days. Nine months is now the maximum wait for any operation, compared with 16 months prior to the project and even outpatient returns are down 45%. The West Midlands RHA has appointed Professor Brian Jarman and Dr Nick Bosanquet of

St Mary's Medical School in London to evaluate the project over the 2-year period.

## Worth Valley

This project also had a 'live' budget and went straight into the scheme without an initial preparatory year in 1994. The Worth Valley Health Consortium is an established sub-committee of Bradford DHA and FHSA and consists of eight practices all of which are fundholding and cover a total population of 60 000 people. The budget is £21 million with management devolved from the Health Authority and with management costs of £134 000 provided by the NHSE plus a further £100 000 from Northern and Yorkshire RHA over 3 years. By going live without a preparatory year, the amount of administrative help required was not fully evaluated and the project manager is now provided with more resources.

The priority for the Consortium is to provide more local services for patients. They hope to do this by turning a former health centre into an intermediate care centre with such out-patient facilities as ultrasound, X-ray and pathology services, but also by providing physiotherapy, occupational therapy and a day centre for the elderly from another site. The Worth Valley Consortium is also predicting savings though as yet the figure is unspecified. An interesting development in Worth Valley is that a member of the social services team is on the project board. This project is to be evaluated by the Nuffield Institute of Health from Leeds.

## Berkshire Integrated Purchasing Project

This project includes 6 fundholding practices and a total of 85 000 patients. The total care budget is about one eighth of the DHA's budget. This amount is based on the proportion of patients in the project compared with the total Berkshire

Health Authority population. This budget is then weighted for any major deviations in age and sex ratios existing between the two populations and possibly also for standard mortality ratio variations.

Agreement was not reached in Berkshire in 1994/5 as to what would happen to any possible savings, but any overspends are to be met from the practices' fundholding savings. There has been excellent co-operation from the Health Authority and the FHSA and the local NHS Trusts.

Information has been a problem but is slowly being collected. The project also introduced pricing sensitive to time spent as an in-patient in 1995/6.

The organizational structure of the project includes a centrally based project manager but each practice validates its own data and runs a notional budget. There has been an agreement that these fundholders do not have to comply with the District strategy but are required to notify the Health Authority when they intend to change their purchasing arrangements. This is most likely to occur in relation to the care of the elderly, whom the Health Authority currently place in private homes. The GPs would prefer to see such patients supported in their own homes. Priorities for the project include geriatric services, hospital transport, midwifery, night centres and extracontractual referrals.

In summary, some of the general objectives of the scheme are to: establish the feasibility of capitation funding; reduce medically inappropriate admissions to hospitals; establish pricing structures that relate prices to length of stay and specific treatment; and rationalize the use of accident and emergency services and the use of non-emergency ambulance provision. Social care is not included in the budget but the relationship with Social Services will be fostered jointly with the Health Authority.

The Health Authority Director of Public Health prepared the specification for the project's evaluation which is being undertaken by the Health Services Management Centre at Birmingham University.

## Castlefields

The fourth project, which went live in 1995/6, is the 'odd man out' and happens to be the project in which I work. The Castlefields Practice in Runcorn with a population of just over 12 000 patients is a single practice total fundholder. This is because there was a feeling within our practice that to have a multi-practice organization would involve a lot of time spent on organizational discussion between the practices, which would slow down the development of the clinical aspects and the public health aspects of the project. The basic premise of this project is that fundholders and Health Authorities have different but complementary skills and by working together in a detailed way will help to harness those skills.

It is possible that this interdependent relationship with the Health Authority will be a more cost-effective approach compared with the other projects and furthermore may well be a model that could be attractive to any political administration. The inherent risk of such a small population is of course in risk management. Work in the USA has suggested that Health Maintenance Organizations needed a population base of at least 50 000 for them to be able to spread the risk if an expensive operation or procedure is necessary. At Castlefields we feel that this risk can be addressed in three ways, none of which has been finalized:

- the Health Authority would pick up the risk in return for the detailed clinical and audit work that we can offer them

- the Health Authority could top slice part of our budget as an insurance scheme

- the Health Authority could offer us a 5-year contract which would enable us in effect to have a 60 000 population.

Preliminary discussions on an unofficial basis with two health economists have suggested that the latter option could be a valid way forward if politically and logistically appropriate.

Future budgets are likely to be based on a needs assessment, partially using as a basis for need the question in the 1991 census relating to chronic health problems. The fact that an estimated million people did not contribute to the census, most of whom were young males, is felt not to affect using such a formula. A needs-based budget can be worked out for every practice in the Health Authority and the actual budget based on that calculation allocated to Castlefields, but obviously not to the other practices in 1995. With this formula, or even on either a historic or a straightforward capitation basis, the Castlefields practice would get a larger budget than it would through fundholding. This confirms the work of Professor Glennester at the London School of Economics, who stated that many of the first and second wave fundholders were underfunded, as their referral patterns and prescribing approaches were more cost-effective than those of many of their colleagues[8].

The project board comprises two doctors from the practice, a project manager who is a joint appointment between the practice and the Health Authority, and whose job also entails working in the Commissioning Team on general commissioning issues for the Health Authority and is the practice's senior manager. Other members of the project team from the Health Authority are the Chief Executive, the Head of Commissioning and the Locality Manager, and a non-executive director. Further board members are the Regional Information Officer and the Regional Fundholding Lead, together with the District Officer for Social Services and a member of the Patients' Health Forum.

The purpose of the project is to explore the effect of the allocation of the total commissioning budget to practice level which could in the future include GMS monies as well as the Health Authority's cash limited allocations. The aims are to:

- develop a model for integrated primary care and local purchasing

- examine the population-based approach to commissioning in a primary care setting

- compare the current referrals patterns and activity basis for the funding of traditional fundholding with a per capita based allocation at a practice level, based on need.

This means identifying the effects, both positive and negative, that a shift to a capitation budget might have at practice level, and exploring the effect that total budget holding at practice level may have on clinical behaviour, both in primary and secondary care settings, for example, the management of 'Did not attends' and hospitalization ratios. It involves evaluating the potential that practice-based total commissioning has for destabilization of strategic commissioning at a population level and defining boundaries of feasible risk management at practice and DHA level and the potential options to deal with these risks. It also involves producing jointly agreed service specifications in order to progress towards joint contract documentation and developing and refining criteria for admission to total practice-based budgets. The following criteria from North Cheshire DHA could be applicable as a prerequisite to other applicants for total budgets:

- integrated management and clinical information systems

- commitment to examine clinical outcomes and to change clinical behaviour

- robust clinical audit systems with evidence of change in practice-based outcome results

- an ability to demonstrate an understanding of risk management and the likely effect on purchasing decisions

- list size of over 10 000 for pilot sites including consortia practices

- ability to demonstrate a commitment to development of the primary health care team ethic

- commitment to and evidence of effective inter-agency collaborative working

- agreement to share a full range of information with the local Health Authority
- demonstrate an effective business management system
- evidence of availability within the practice of appropriate management skills or commitment to ensure they are recruited
- willingness to agree to Health Authority participation in any recruitment of staff for the project
- evidence of user input into service development within the practice
- established quality assurance programme in the practice
- agreement to work to project plan and report progress as set out in the plan
- agreement to regular meetings with the project board and nominated key liaison officer from the DHA and a non-executive director of the Health Authority
- agreement to contribute to and work within the local Health Authority strategic framework developing innovative approaches to service developments
- ability to disseminate good practice and influence peers.

The key innovations expected at the Castlefields practice are listed below.

- A model for maternity care which by April 1996 will integrate community-based and hospital-based midwifery for a practice population.

- A reduction in emergency admissions using hospital-at-home, and the auditing of accident and emergency staff behaviour and general practice behaviour, offering the GP as a possible second opinion for the junior admitting staff if a patient is felt to need admission from Casualty attendance. Research evidence suggests that 15% of emergency surgical admissions could be avoided if patients were seen by a senior hospital doctor on arrival at the hospital. We want to change that approach by utilizing the on-call GP when patients are attending the Casualty Unit.

- A utilization review model for in-patients using the project manager for such assessment (similar to work already described at Bromsgrove where the visiting nurse liaison officer suggests alternative packages of care for in-patients).

- Reducing hospital follow-up visits to a minimum.

- Minimizing those investigations being done in hospitals, which could be carried out or at least organized within primary care.

- Employing a mental illness care manager for patients registered with the practice, even if much of their care is secondary-setting oriented.

Much of this work is an extension of fundholding, as the Castlefields practice always held the view that the chief purpose of being a fundholding practice was to have a primary care budget from which cost-effective care for patients would be developed. Total fundholding has increased the scope and responsibility of the fundholding scheme, which will be a more exciting yet exacting challenge for both the general practice and the Health Authority as a result.

A further innovation is to include the GMS budget in the total practice budget and track progress. Legally GPs have still to be paid in the traditional way and therefore this has to be an indicative approach at the present time.

GPs have traditionally regarded GMS monies as being 'their money'. As recently highlighted by Plamping and Fischer in the *Health Services Journal*[9], GMS should be regarded as a resource for the GP's practice population out of which GPs are paid. To this end total fundholding and GMS monies should combine to be a total resource available for the practice population. The more components in a budget, the more equitable the setting of that budget. This point was demonstrated by work undertaken at York University exploring whether or not traditional fundholding could be capitation based. The work for the NHSE suggested that since fundholding only takes into account some of the total primary care health resource, an equitable budget was almost impossible based solely on capitation. The total budget as described at Castlefields is moving towards such an equitable provision, especially as in the North Cheshire model the budget is based on an overall needs assessment.

The evaluation of the Castlefields project is being undertaken by Professor Margaret Pearson of the Health and Community Care Research Unit, Liverpool University, and is to compare purchasing and commissioning at a practice level with the activities undertaken at Health Authority level.

# Looking to the future

In February 1995, action was undertaken by the NHSE to support the further total fundholding initiative by the provision of facilitation support (with a further major conference) and further evaluation arrangements as follows.

## Facilitation support

An assessment is to be made for each site, of the progress made to date and the future programme of work. A development programme is to set out recommendations on the scope of any facilitation support required for the overall national evaluation, with proposals on how the programme is to be taken forward.

## Evaluation

The NHSE wish to evaluate the total purchasing pilots in order to learn and inform further planning and implementation of this initiative. To ensure independent external evaluation a consortium of seven research institutes, coordinated by the King's Fund College in London, is undertaking this exercise. The aims of the evaluation are to assess the costs and benefits attributable to the extension of GP fundholding to total purchasing. The evaluation is therefore focusing on the implementation and impact of the pilot schemes to obtain research-based evidence on:

- the factors associated with successful set up and operation of total purchasing

- the costs and effectiveness of total purchasing

- the benefits to patients of total purchasing.

Some of the key issues which the evaluation will address are discussed below.

### Operation of pilot schemes

The evaluation over the 1995/6 period should describe the process of implementation of the schemes covering such aspects as:

- the role of the Health Authority in terms of managerial and organizational support

- the administrative work-load for the practices

- resource inputs, including time, skills and technological infrastructure

- information and IT requirements

- formal arrangements to involve all practices in decisions on contracting use of savings and provider configuration

- the process of budget setting

- health needs assessments
- arrangements for contracting
- arrangements for management of risk
- accountability arrangements.

### Costs of total purchasing
The evaluation will include operating costs, transaction costs, efforts to minimize costs, budget management, overhead spends and underspends, and use of savings.

### Effectiveness of total purchasing
The evaluation should assess:

- prescribing patterns
- referral and investigation patterns
- consultation on purchasing plans
- quality in contracts; the balance of service provision at primary and secondary interface and provider configuration; and variations from both Health Authority purchasing strategy and national priorities.

### Benefits to patients
The benefits to patients should focus on responsiveness to patient choices and how the operation of the pilot schemes affects waiting times and access to primary and secondary care. Health outcomes associated with purchasing management should also be studied as well as the impact on delivery of general medical services in the pilot sites.

### Services requiring special focus and evaluation
Services requiring special focus and evaluation include: emergency admission and accident and emergency; mental health and services for people with learning disabilities; maternity services; community care; palliative care; regional specialties and health promotion.

## Best models

To evaluate the best models for the further development of fundholding based purchasing in a primary care led NHS elements of good practice in total purchasing should be identified. In relation to patient populations, the relationship of practice participants to a complete geographical locality and coverage of health services and specialties need to be studied.

## Design and methods of evaluation

Sites for the national pilot are, of course, volunteer practices which have been selected through a collaborative process. Random assignment cannot therefore be part of the design of the evaluation. A research design in which total purchasing can be assessed in comparison with a mixed economy of standard fundholding and DHA purchasing would further enhance the scientific standing and credibility of the evaluation. Given the scale of this total purchasing initiative, it has been suggested that it would not seem appropriate to conduct the evaluation in the same degree of depth in relation to all the sites. Therefore a two level approach with a collection of a standardized body of data across all sites and more intensive investigation of a small number of selected sites is to be carried out. The methodology suggested comprises analysis of time-series data, documentary analysis, structured and semi-structured interviews, surveys, observation of process, case studies of critical incident and problem management. An initial phase of evaluation should include at least an assessment of the available database in relation to the information requirements; discussion with pilot sites and with key stakeholders about their objectives and priorities regarding the total practice purchasing scheme; and establishing links with the locally appointed researchers of the four existing total purchasing pilot sites. The evaluation will be expected to prepare a first interim report 6 months after the start of the research project, a second interim report 12 months from the start and a final report on completion.

# Summing up

Primary care budgets may be the way forward for a more responsive devolved NHS. The question is whether or not general practice as an organization is up to this task? My feelings are that general practice or any other primary care organization based on practice populations must demonstrate skills and commitment to:

* needs assessment

* clinical resource management

* practice population commissioning.

British general practice is unusual in having a registered population of patients. The practice can therefore be a truly managed care organization, providing services where appropriate and to paraphrase the words of Barry Robinson of Lyme Regis Community Unit 'Purchasing services which it cannot provide' (*see* p. 204). Health needs assessment is essential to ensure a local budget is responsive to need. The Castlefields model of needs assessment involves the following approaches.

* Use of IT so that a paperless practice system based on computers can ensure excellent audit, but even more important build up a morbidity database.

* Community feedback through contacts with local Councillors, through community development work, through patient surveys and through a local health forum.

* A public health approach using various techniques, such as rapid appraisal and epidemiology to identify other unmet needs in the community, whether it be disease based or other health problem areas. The practice can have a true commissioning role in either providing services, purchasing services or commissioning other organizations to meet the identified need.

- A social care project which involves a care manager undertaking the primary health care team assessment of social care needs and helping to identify packages of care to meet such needs through a locally devolved budget.

- This work is described in detail elsewhere[10,11]. The other area of responsibility for the primary care team is that of a clinical resource management. The GP, whether as a lead person in the primary care organization, as in the current models of primary care, or as the lead clinical person in any other primary care organization, needs to ensure that the clinical resource is appropriately used.

In the Castlefields practice we challenged our own clinical behaviour and can show evidence of change of clinical behaviour through audit. We have also set contracts with secondary care clinicians to ensure clinical guideline setting and audit[11,12]. We have purchased for protocols and audit and have moved contracts on clinical grounds following either audit or a review of clinical effectiveness or appropriateness. We have only changed contracts following clinical discussions, but in some cases have needed to move the contract as a lever to achieve clinical behaviour change. This approach should be reliant on evidence-based medicine where available. The GP has a key role in ensuring that clinical procedures are appropriate for patients. In the past, general practice, when referring to secondary care has tended to cede responsibility to the secondary care providers. The new role for the GP is to be the clinical care manager for patients, whether they are being looked after by primary care, in shared care or almost totally being looked after in secondary care. This care management approach will ensure that cost-effective responsive treatment is being offered.

Many people, including GPs, have criticized fundholding as interfering with the advocacy role of general practice. That advocacy role seems to me to be a very narrow approach, where advocacy relates to whether a patient is to be referred to secondary care in the traditional gate-keeper function. Fundholding can enhance advocacy by ensuring that inappropriate medical activity or ineffective medical activity is curtailed, and furthermore by responding to needs based on a practice population.

The new NHS will develop further when we have more explicit accountability. The NHS has been traditionally a command and control model, always demanding accountability to the tier above. To ensure sufficient tension in the system and yet co-operation, I would suggest a very explicit two tier accountability to the tier above and to the tier below the organization. To this end, general practice needs to be much more explicitly accountable to its practice population not only via the individual consultation but furthermore by such models as patient councils, patient forums, patient participation groups or utilizing the Community Health Councils. A practice should also be explicitly accountable to the local Health Authority, as at Castlefields, where we have set standards on clinical care, patient access, organizational standards and exploring a social science methodology to demonstrate the quality of our non-clinical care. This accountability framework could be the model for how GP and Primary Health Care Team members are to be remunerated.

Health Authorities should be accountable through corporate contracts to their regional office of the NHSE but equally need to be much more explicitly accountable to GPs whether fundholders or not. Provider units too should expect quality standards from the GPs and in particular fundholders. Two-way contracts for ensuring quality and responsiveness are all deliverable in this framework. Primary care led purchasing in total fundholding mode, with such accountability could well lead to an NHS not split into a bureaucratic provider and purchasing approach, but to general practice as the deliverer of managed care to ensure cost-effective approaches in response to identified needs.

In this model, the Health Authority will be a facilitator of primary care but would expect explicit standards to be delivered. The division between primary, secondary and even tertiary care will be increasingly blurred as best packages of care are developed defining what standards of care should be set and only then developing approaches to decide where care should be delivered and by whom. The ultimate responsibility for this needs to be with the primary care budget holder. I would expect, as the relationship between Health Authorities and GPs matures, that intelligent decisions would be made as to where purchasing should take place. For high technology, high cost, low volume services, the purchasing should be at least at the level of the Health Authority if not beyond. For instance, this could be by an agency for many Health Authorities, but even within Health Authority and GP interfaces, different decisions about who has the purchasing skills would have to be made at local level. This imaginative decision-making takes honesty, imagination and trust and total fundholding could be the development model to induce such development. Total fundholding provides an essential development beyond traditional fundholding to develop an NHS which is both devolved and local and yet still a national service. This approach will or should be party political proof, founded on evidence-based activity delivered locally through clear accountability.

Total fundholding has obvious advantages over traditional fundholding, in that the budgets will be seen to be set equitably. GPs will have strategic responsibility as well as accountability to the individual, and should demonstrate, as suggested by Roberts *et al* 'that NHS funding is sufficient to avoid any need to deny effective health care for the foreseeable future. The problem is not insufficient funds but poor management which is failing to direct money where it is needed most. Accepting explicit rationing now would institutionalize current inefficiencies and neutralize any future attempt at correction. The main obstacle to change and therefore to the salvation of the NHS as we know it are the workforces' cultural resistance, vested interests, weak management and frequent political interference'[13].

I am suggesting that primary care led purchasing in particular through total fundholding with increased accountability, could help to tackle such obstacles, working always in complementary conjunction with Health Authorities.

# References

1  Carruthers I (1994) Total fundholding in the mainstream of the NHS. *Primary Care Management.* **4**: 7–9.

2  National Health Service Executive (1994) EL(94)79 *Developing NHSE purchasing and general practice fundholding.* NHSE, London.

3  National Health Service Executive (1993) *New world, new opportunities.* NHSE, London.

4  Anon (1994) The fundholding summary. *Times Health Supplement.*

5  Society *The Guardian.* 25 January 1995.

6  Fundholding Bulletin. *Haymarket Medical,* 7 December 1994.

7  National Health Service Executive (1995) *Purchasing in practice.* NHSE, London, Issue 2.

8  Glennester H *et al.* (1993) Wild card or winning hand? In: Robinson R and Le Grand J (eds), *Evaluating the NHS reforms.* King's Fund Institute, London, pp. 74–197.

9  Plamping D and Fischer M (1994) Family values. *Health Service J.* **104**: 22–3.

10  Colin-Thomé D (1994) Practice population commissioning. In: Peel V, Sheaffe R and Higgins J (eds) *Best practice in healthcare commissioning.* Longman, Harlow.

11  Colin-Thomé D (1994) Commissioning, purchasing and planning. In: Rea C (ed) *Managing clinical directorates.* Longman, Harlow.

12  Colin-Thomé D (1995) Future development. In: Henry S and Pickersgill D (eds) *Making sense of fundholding.* Radcliffe Medical Press, Oxford. pp. 199–208.

13  Roberts C *et al.* (1995) Rationing is a desperate measure. *Health Services J.* **105**: 15.

# The preferred provider    | 5

*Nigel Sylvester*

Mother NHS could always be relied on. She was always there to scoop you off the pavement, free at the point of delivery, universal, caring and all knowing. It was a pleasant warm feeling knowing that there were always plump ruddy nurses and clever doctors to make us better when we grazed our knees. However, we have grown up now and She has been confronted by a more mature group of patients. Exposed as inconsistent, wasteful, self-deluding and sometimes incompetent, those moments of compassion and brilliance often seem submerged by an over confidence that She 'had it right'.

Now we are left with a more brutally honest NHS; an NHS that has to account for itself; that has to justify the huge amounts of taxpayers' money it consumes; that has to explain why patients die more readily in certain hospitals; and at last has to listen to an adult population who have been patronized for too long.

What are the responses to this muscular NHS? Patients are encouraged by an antagonistic press to feel insecure; worry that their hospital is going to be closed down; that their treatment is cheap and ineffective; and when they need it most, that a manager is going to bar their entry to salvation. No matter how many hands are held and graphs shown, a single shroud waved from an upper window of a Victorian mental asylum by a white-haired consultant frightens us all into thinking that She was not so bad after all. The medical profession has responded to the new NHS with a range of emotional reactions; enthusiasm from those who believe that doctors should be involved in health care organization to hostility from those who believe it taints their art.

The huge loss of public confidence caused by political games and the apparent obsession with the language of the market place must be restored by a clearly understood message that the patients are getting a better deal.

It is clear that in addition to a huge commitment of patient care, those who believe in the reforms have another task. It has to be demonstrated that what has been done to the NHS is not just random matricide but a scientific, well-considered change for the better. This can only be done when all purchasers, fundholders, non-fundholders, Commissions, Health Authorities and Consortia work to an identifiable strategy that can demonstrate health gain. The enormous difference this time around is that the strategy is informed by the patient's advocate, the GP.

This change means that new relationships will have to develop between the new integrated Health Authorities or Commissions and their primary care co-purchasers. Indeed, Commissions may wish to, or have to, devolve the majority of purchasing to primary care which will become 'providers' of a surrogate purchasing mechanism. Those who embrace this role and can demonstrate proficiency will become the preferred providers. Indeed these practices or groups of practices can become purchasers for all care, replacing a major role of the pre-1996 DHA.

## The role of the Health Commissions

Assuming parliamentary assent, the merged authorities (FHSAs and DHAs) will gain legal status in April 1996. The resulting slimmed down Health Authority should be a much more efficient organ to develop primary care. The GMS functions of the FHSA and the purchasing functions of the old DHAs will be brought together under the same roof. The posture they adopt over delegating purchasing will be critical to the success of primary care development. There are four essential ingredients.

## Purchasing strategy

It is widely acknowledged that decisions affecting patient care should be devolved down to the point of patient contact. Decisions on clinical matters, staff deployment and physical infrastructure should rightly be made where the daily dilemmas are most acutely felt. Certainly the central command-and-control model which hitherto has resulted in paralysis of initiative, misinvestment and demoralization has had its day.

The new role of Health Commissions is well laid out in the NHSE document EL(94)79[1]. They are encouraged to decrease their direct purchasing role in favour of a strategic, monitoring and support function. The broad view that a Commission has to take in relation to the planning of coherent and relatively homogeneous services across a large area requires a strategy to which all purchasers in that area can subscribe. This obviously requires a dialogue between GP purchasers and Commission planners.

Early in the reforms the North and Mid-Hampshire Health Commission recognized, in the area where I practice, that developing purchasing strategies is a two-way process. Accordingly, it was recognized that to purchase in an integrated and intelligent way GPs need to understand:

• what the Commission's priorities are and why

• what the collateral effects of investment shifts are likely to be

• what financial parameters they are working within

- what quality issues are paramount

- what the attitude to honest investment errors is going to be.

Similarly the Commission needs to understand about GPs:

- what their purchasing priorities are and why

- what their long-term aspirations are for their patients (and whether their patients have been consulted)

- what the delivery of quality standards is like

- whether purchasing shifts are going to occur and why.

Many GPs are wary of an overbearing authority reducing their freedom to purchase what they like, when they like, with whom they like. However, too many wild cards can endanger providers that satisfy the majority of purchasers. Commissions may wish to invest in a service that requires commitment from GPs to a purchasing strategy for it to succeed. A strategy that is informed by as many GP purchasers as possible has a much greater chance of success than the top down approach of old. Understanding the above factors helps this process.

This shared ownership of a strategy has to start early in the contracting cycle if there is to be any chance of success. The Commission's ideas have to be flagged early for the GPs to respond and similarly the GPs must have their plans well thought out before any purposeful dialogue can take place. Formulation of a 5-year plan by Commissions enables joint planning to be even better informed and gives an opportunity to all parties, including Community Health Councils, and other organizations to shape local health care appropriately.

In the future, GPs are likely to take on most purchasing. It is therefore incumbent on them now to take a greater responsibility for strategic development, lest they be accused of having their cake and eating it.

## Monitoring and support

Now NHSE regional offices have devolved monitoring to Commissions there must be a clear understanding what the parameters are and what sanctions are to be brought to bear if purchasers fall outside those parameters. The NHSE guidance on fundholding accountability gives some guidelines[2] but it is still important that local agreements are clear on what is acceptable and what is not. The issue of the use of savings, particularly in the face of longer-than-average waiting times, is an example of a possible source of conflict, where GPs need clear guidance.

Support for the Commissions' co-purchasers will also become progressively more important. Crucially, Commissions must encourage the development of purchasing groups that represent all practices in a given area, non-fundholding and fundholding alike. Although fundholding groups have been successful in independently organizing themselves, there is a strong case for Commissions to encourage their effectiveness through clerical support and the provision of liaison members. Obviously purely non-fundholding groups and GP commissioning groups would benefit in the same way. The Winchester Purchasing Group has been operating successfully since 1991 with fundholders, non-fundholders and Commission representatives meeting every 6 weeks. The sharing of tasks such as the creation of a common quality standard has been a relatively easy task and has reduced suspicion that one group is being favoured over another.

Although the central command model has failed, a headlong rush to the other pole could lead to as many idiosyncratic decisions being made under the laudable but so far untested, thesis that 'near is best'. There is an obvious danger of practices with particular interests, or more importantly disinterests, causing holes in a poorly managed system at the district level. So far there is no evidence this is occurring, but with successive waves of less enthusiastic purchasers coming into the system this will become an increasing danger. The danger was increased in 1995 by the political imperative which forced NHS regional offices to seek out further waves of fundholders who may not be up to the job. Disaster looms if incompetent fundholders take over the important purchasing roles of competent Health Authorities. The Commissions which adopt a positive attitude to strategy, monitoring and support will help avoid these potential sources of dislocation in the service.

## Probity and fairness

For the new NHS to earn the trust of the public its financial arrangements must be completely transparent and open to scrutiny. It must be clearly shown that individual doctors cannot benefit from the system and that their motivation to be a part of the reformed NHS is improvement in patient care alone.

The apparent inequity of access to service makes the system vulnerable to ill-informed attack. The variations in service must be demonstrated to be variations in priority of the purchaser and inequality of the populations they serve rather than an inequity in the service.

Equity and equality are not the same. It is axiomatic that a practice population with a large number of elderly dependent patients should have a greater access to a service than a young relatively athletic practice population. The access therefore depends on need rather than a head count. Needs assessment is an important science that must be developed so that it is integrated into the budget-setting process. The apparent inequity of provision that the providers perceive can only be justified if a difference in population requirements has been demonstrated. This has obviously not been possible so far and in some areas of the country has caused distrust between non-fundholders and their fundholding colleagues.

In North and Mid-Hampshire a framework for co-operation between fundholders, non-fundholders and the Commission has been in existence since 1993. Constructed with the intention of publicly demonstrating a firm commitment to process (eg non-fundholding consortia etc), it has helped to reduce suspicion that one group is being favoured over another.

The framework is laid out in a document: *The future direction of fundholding*[3] and is summarized into the following 10 principles.

- Fundholders should be considered as co-purchasers alongside the Commission's 'in house' purchasing teams.

- Fundholders must be able to retain their flexibility as small purchasers while working alongside the Commission and must be able to experiment.

- The Commission will actively support the development and expansion of fundholding; alternative models of practice-based purchasing will be evaluated.

- The funding policy for fundholding needs to ensure openness and fairness in the allocation and use of resources.

- The standard public expenditure criteria of probity and value for money apply equally to the Commission and fundholders.

- The pattern of services purchased by the Commission and purchased and provided by fundholders needs to be consistent with national and regional objectives and standards.

- Purchasers and providers have a mutual interest in looking to the longer term.

- Fundholders and the Commission need to take a shared view of the best use of resources available to the Commission each year.

- Information and intelligence about commissioning should be shared and publicly reported.

- The money spent on direct patient care should be maximized.

These principles have underpinned a determination to demonstrate that the fundholders are not being preferentially treated.

## Purchasing quality standards

Purchasing has, to date, largely revolved around driving waiting times down. Already by 1995, many purchasers reached the point where waiting times are of less pressing importance. Purchasing higher quality standards is becoming of greater significance. This quality drive can be divided into scientific quality (ie effectiveness) and service quality (ie delivery).

### Scientific quality
Scientific quality can be defined as those parts of our purchasing that are based on evidence of efficacy. There is a huge amount of medical practice based on out-of-date information. The difference in survival rates in hospitals with similar populations for certain cancers is a potent indication of this. (Outdated practice continues in primary care but is a separate issue.) There is, however, considerable scope for purchasers to apply pressures for change across a wide range of less dramatic activity. Most purchasing to date has been on the basis of trust and while this is often well placed it is now incumbent on purchasers to ensure best practice is being employed.

It must be recognized however, that 'best practice' may be more expensive. Purchasers are rarely given information on methods and materials used, as this has always been the preserve of consultant staff. However, there may be situations when, if given sufficient information, a purchaser might opt for an expensive option for long-term gain. For example, if a certain variety of hip replacement is shown in most research to be best in given situations, then those replacements should be used even if there is pressure to keep costs as low as possible.

At present, purchasers do not have sufficient knowledge to challenge current practice and therefore may be ignorantly purchasing suboptimal treatment. Effectiveness bulletins, produced by careful research in Leeds[4] and other centres, are an important tool in this process. The evaluation of techniques from all available sources now gives the purchaser a more informed view of what he or she wishes to buy. Some fundholders have even refused to pay for out-dated management. An example of this is in the treatment of premature labour. There is now incontrovertible evidence that mothers in preterm labour should receive steroids to reduce the incidence of respiratory distress in pre-term infants. Fundholders are now refusing to pay for treatment that does not include such management.

As purchasing becomes more scientific the major advantage Commissions have over GPs is a huge capacity to process information. Health Authorities' Public Health Consultants have all the necessary skills to interpret such information and to determine its local applicability. In the meantime, practices such as our own in Winchester will purchase the time of consultants in public health to process this information and determine its local relevance. It is obviously a time-consuming business and risks duplication of effort.

### Service quality

Service quality can be defined as those contracted and measurable features of delivery that directly impact on the patients' welfare. These include waiting times, return to theatre rates, death within one month of operation rates and infection rates. Many purchasers, particularly fundholders, have been hammering away at these from the beginning of the NHS reforms. There is now software available that can collate information from a range of providers on these indices, and others, such as costs. Purchasers can and should incorporate information requirements into contracts, which after processing, can be passed onto other purchasers to inform their contracting next time round.

The advent of effectiveness bulletins and better surveillance of service delivery is, therefore, an important stage in the drive towards intelligent purchasing by GPs. The synthesis of detailed reliable information from providers (eg outcome measures), and well-researched effectiveness information should ultimately bring about a credible assessment of what 'best practice' is available to a purchaser in a given locality and whether it is being employed as widely as it should be.

## The preferred provider

It is a commonly held view that Commissions are too remote from the patient to be sensitive enough to the wishes of the population they serve. However great their efforts to consult the public and gather intelligence on provider efficiency there will always be a separation between them and the populations they serve that will be impossible to straddle. What further complicates the issue is that Commissions are often paying for care rather than purchasing it. While Commissions may put into place contracts that deliver the required health care in a given locality, they are in fact usually only formalizing an arrangement to pay for the care that GPs have, in effect, decided to purchase. Contracts therefore usually follow referral flow rather than lead it.

It seems logical that demand for a service and the purchase of that service come from the same agency. An agency, therefore that provides a service of extended primary care and the effective arrangement of residual secondary care is arguably preferable to the division that has always applied. A general practice purchaser can thereby expand its role to be the designated local preferred provider of all care.

Currently, when purchasing decisions are made, a provider is normally awarded a service agreement with a purchaser because of a number of factors. They include proximity, historic association, demonstrable quality, ability to change and cost benefit. These factors are relatively easy to assess for the purchaser of elective care, but the extension into other areas of purchasing requires considerably greater sophistication than that previously undertaken. The key feature that primary care can instil into the new contracts is a flexibility which enables the release of initiative.

In future, the purchaser will consider quality more critically. The transfer of the majority of purchasing to primary care must be invested in groups who can develop systems that have the same critical analysis capabilities as the Commissions.

At Friarsgate in Winchester, we expect experiments in total fundholding to expose the weaknesses in this shift, and provide GPs with enormous experience for improving the way they can deliver a wider range of better care.

# Prerequisites for the devolution of purchasing to primary care

## Accreditation

There is a huge inconsistency in standards in primary care. The medical profession has managed to protect the mediocre and poor providers of care by maintaining that clinical freedom should always be paramount in the relationship between patient and doctor. Sloppy thinking has therefore been able to masquerade as something virtuous whilst patients' interests have been neglected. For primary care to be the focus of health care provision there must be a robust accreditation system in place to ensure patients are getting a good quality service. Unless this is taken up by the profession with greater vigour it will be imposed in a manner the profession finds less palatable. Notable among these options could be very restrictive practice-based contracts which would enable commissioning authorities to impose standards as a prerequisite for continuing financial support. The GMSC is making useful progress in this aim but will be met by elements within the profession which feel that they should be allowed to practice in whatever way they like, despite being public servants spending public money.

## Organizational capacity

In order to maximize income, because of its independent contractor status, general practice has always had a major interest in organizing itself efficiently. The basic principles of financial and personnel management are therefore integral to GP training. However, the scale or organization required for devolved purchasing is of a different order. There must be a recognition of doctors' limitations in management skills and the acceptance that expensive skills will have to be brought in. This element must be examined carefully in the assessment of the cost benefits of the proposed change.

## Rationing

If primary care is to accept the role of preferred provider it will have to accept some of the difficult responsibility of arbiter in rationing decisions. GPs have always rationed resources although these decisions have never been explicit. There are a wide range of rationing decisions GPs make at present. These range from the rationing of time afforded to each patient to the gate-keeper role guarding scarce secondary resources. Decisions about difficult issues, such as the availability of *in vitro* fertilization will inevitably follow devolved purchasing. This will lead to the conflict of representing the best interests of the community over the interests of individual patients. For doctors, who are trained to take a focused, individual-centred view this will create new stresses. Community perspectives will inevitably intrude into this relationship and some may find that cultural shift too great. General practice will have to accommodate these responsibilities by consulting with local groups and public health consultants about which areas of spending have to be restrained. However, when these decisions are made, they must always be prefaced by an acknowledgement that deficient central funding is the source of the dilemma rather than a perverse desire to deprive patients of services they want. These debates will be more painful in primary care than to Health Authorities as they will be confronted by their own rationing decisions every day.

## Accountability

The fundholding accountability framework referred to above[2] is reasonable if the public can be assured that the NHS has high standards that are properly managed by the overseeing authorities. However, probity and minimum national standards apart, the framework must not be seen as a way of corralling general practices into adopting a purchasing strategy that they do not co-own. The preferred provider's responsibilities for integrating care will permit a much more mature relationship with overseeing authorities or regulators.

# Conclusion

If primary care is to move centre stage and become a provider of all care by providing high quality primary care and buying in all secondary care on behalf of Health Authorities it must demonstrate it can do the task in a well researched and co-ordinated manner using the best available information and management skills. For it to deliver better care to the public it must listen to the population it serves and liaise effectively with all others who have an interest in the health of that population. It is a huge task, but one well worth taking on, the prize of success is too important to lose. Those GPs who succeed will be the preferred providers of the future.

# References

1   National Health Service Executive (1994) EL (94)79. *Developing NHS purchasing and GP fundholding.* NHSE, London.

2   National Health Service Executive (1995) EL (95) 54. *Accountability framework for GP fundholding.* NHSE, London.

3   North & Mid-Hampshire Health Authority (1993) *The future direction of fundholding* (unpublished).

4   Health Care Effective Bulletins. (1992–1995) Nuffield Institute, Leeds.

# The general practice Consortium: the future of fundholding?

6

*Hugh Maclean*

## The formation of the Isle of Wight Consortium

In 1992, there was widespread dissatisfaction amongst local GPs with the quality of the contracts negotiated by the island's Health Authority. The increasing ability of first- and second-wave fundholding practices to negotiate preferential access to services created an environment of uncertainty among many of the non-fundholding GPs. This led in turn to a growing awareness of a need for change. Two parallel local studies were initiated, looking at possible routes to purchasing. One study examined the possible implications of 'shadow (or indicative) fundholding' and the other looked at full fundholding.

The first study looked at how GPs could influence the contracting process by influencing the decisions of the DHA, yet avoiding the administrative problems involved in running full fundholding. The drawback seemed to be the difficulty of gaining accurate activity data as this would be based only on information from providers. Thus, there would have to be at least some data collection at practice level. It seemed likely that 'shadow' fundholding would involve nearly as much work as full fundholding if it was to succeed. Additionally there was the difficulty in funding the extra work required of GPs, their staff and the Isle of Wight Health Commission managers, as the financial resources would have to come from existing Commission budgets. Another problem was the lack of a guaranteed return of any savings made. The Health Commission was obliged to balance its own budget year on year and this would take priority over making payments to practices achieving savings.

The second study looked at entering fundholding as a co-operative. We would adopt a common purchasing approach, and present a strong unified face to the providers. This, it was hoped, would reduce the number of individual negotiations the provider unit had to go through to finalize its contracts. We also wished to maintain equity of access to services for all island patients, and avoid any suggestion of a two-tier service. Improvements would, wherever possible, be made available to fundholders and non-fundholders alike. The approach also allowed maximum flexibility for practices to develop individually tailored contracts as well as formulating joint quality specifications and common contracts where appropriate. Another issue that we wished to address was that of having a single island provider. It would be easy for the actions of a significant number of fundholders to damage services seriously. If this threatened the viability of acute services to the island's population then the continuation of fundholding would be able to predict those actions that would cause problems to the provider and avoid them.

An extraordinary meeting of the Local Medical Committee reviewed both options in the early autumn of 1992. It decided that both methods of purchasing were likely to require substantial amounts of work by participating practices and consequently the independence of full fundholding seemed a more sensible route. A team of interested GPs was elected to take the matter forward. After negotiations with the Health Commission and the Wessex RHA, eight funds were approved. Three funds were awarded to single practices large enough to hold funds on their own and five funds went to pairs of smaller practices, making a total of 13 practices, with eight funds. A centralized management structure was formulated, with each fund contributing a share of its management allowance to pay the expenses of staffing and running the central office.

The Island Health Care Consortium is now the result of this large group of GPs from the Isle of Wight combining together to become fourth-wave fundholders. In 1995, the Island has a population of 128 000 with some 65 000 patients looked after by the 12 practices remaining in the Consortium and a further 38 000 looked after by four other first- and second-wave fundholders.

This group was accepted into the preparatory year from April 1993 and spent the next six months gathering activity data. This material was reconciled with information from the providers to set the budgets that would apply once the practices went live from April 1994. Fundholding software and IT requirements were investigated and suppliers chosen. Although the product selected has generally performed as expected, support from the supplier has been less than we would have wished.

Autumn 1993 saw the appearance in practices of another innovation, the Practice Health Plan. This involved each practice in an enormous amount of work, as it had to contain information about:

- the practice
- its staff and their duties
- its surgery facilities
- its patient profile and demography
- its major health needs and priorities for the next 12 months
- any developments foreseen in the next year.

September 1993 also saw the publication of the Consortium's Common Quality Standards document, which laid down the basis for the contracts we would be negotiating with our providers. This was generally well received and gave clear and informed assistance to the creation of the Island Health Commission's own quality standard document.

Many other subjects had to be considered during this period, including:

- the Consortium Membership Agreement

- cluster agreements

- whether Consortium member practices would have to be combined in clusters

- whether small practices within Consortia should be able to hold practice-based funds.

The last point is important, because it became evident that practices were widely different in their funding requirements. This has now become the focus of negotiations with the Department of Health, and in 1996 we are still hoping for a change in the regulations.

By December 1993, the activity information from practices was being reconciled with that from the main providers, and initial budget offers began to appear from the RHA in early March. Contract negotiations began with our main providers on the Isle of Wight, and also with two new providers from the mainland.

As March 1994 approached, we unfortunately lost one practice from the Consortium as they had concerns over the effect that fundholding would have on their practice policies for prescribing and dispensing. The effect of this was to leave their cluster partner unable to continue as a fundholder, unless paired with another practice. This was a blow, as we lost £35 000 of management allowance as a result. It was only through the generosity of member practices and the help of the FHSA that we managed to move the other practice to another cluster within the Consortium. We did, however, gain from the merger of a single-handed practice with one of our member practices. This left us representing some 65 000 patients, about 50% of the Island's population. If other fundholders are taken into account, then 85% of the island's patients were, in 1995, looked after by fundholding practices. This compares with the current South and West regional average of 32% and the national average of 35% for 1994/5.

This group of 12 practices was accepted for fourth-wave fundholding from April 1994 and now functions under the title of the Island Health Care Consortium. Since its inception the co-operative spirit that has developed within the Consortium has helped doctors, managers and practice staff alike. This can only benefit patients as access to care becomes easier.

## Organization

Figure 1 illustrates the working of our Consortium. Each member practice (irrespective of size) elects one voting member onto the Consortium board. The board meets monthly and is responsible for the strategy and policy of the Consortium. An executive is appointed from the board at the annual general meeting by all GPs in the Consortium, not just by

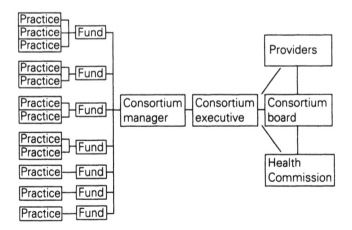

**Figure 1**  Organization.

members of the Board. The executive, along with the general manager and his staff have the responsibility for ensuring that the decisions of the Board are put into effect.

## Why the Consortium approach?

We chose a consortium approach in 1993 for the following reasons.

- There was a need to influence standards of secondary care, without destabilizing our single hospital provider.

- We wished to rationalize the multiple negotiations that would arise if many more practices were to go fundholding.

- We wanted to unite the contracting and administrative functions under a high quality manager (beyond the resources of a single fund).

- We wanted to set up a support network for practices and to obtain economies of scale that would result in higher quality purchasing decisions.

- We wanted to be able to move some services into the primary care sector, when appropriate, which can be difficult for individual fundholders to achieve.

- We wished to make best use of the resources offered in the management fund, and to use it to maximize the benefit to the member practices.

- We wanted to reduce the workload on GPs.

- We wished to be in a position to protect our single acute provider and it is easier in a Consortium/multi-fund arrangement to consider the long-term effects of significant changes in our purchasing strategy.

### Advantages of a Consortium
Our analysis of the benefits of this approach in 1995 shows that a Consortium can be responsible for purchasing and commis-

sioning services for a wider population enabling a coherent approach to developments.

The support networks of a Consortium offer efficiency gains for members specifically:

• the system of lead GPs in purchasing means fewer hours lost from the provision of primary care

• Practice Managers' Groups have developed information and support networks at practice administration level

• the Consortium management is able to provide wider support to practices than pure fundholding with further spin-offs including training in wordprocessing, spreadsheet working and management techniques.

The Consortium is able to protect the individuality of practices. Practices need to be able to keep their identities. One of the great strengths of general practice is its diversity, and this is not threatened by being members of a Consortium.

The independent contractor status of GPs is a long-standing right, which is enshrined in the original National Health Act of 1948. The independence issue remains important today. We have developed a strong and successful primary care service in the UK because general practice has remained outside the control of the secondary care sector. In countries where hospitals are the prime focus for care, costs are higher and quality is often inferior. Here, because the profession has been responsible for delivering primary care, quality of service has steadily improved and the standing of general practice within the medical profession has been dramatically raised. It is from this background that the concept of purchasing primary care has grown. Health Commissions are seen as needing to gain greater control over the clinical freedoms of GPs and these freedoms will not willingly be given up. It is only where there is some mutual advantage that co-operation is likely to be forthcoming. As a result, the worry that the existence of large aggregates of practices will threaten the competitive nature of general practice is likely to be unfounded.

Our experience on the Isle of Wight is that, where there is a mutual advantage in using common contracts, this will be the route that GPs will follow. However, if there is an advantage for one practice to put in place a service that is not shared by neighbouring practices, then there is nothing inherent in a Consortium or multi-fund concept that prevents this. The independent nature of GPs will generally mean that innovation will continue, and certainly our Consortium has no wish to stifle development, as long as it does not disadvantage the patients of others.

A Consortium also addresses locality issues effectively because practices can combine with neighbours to purchase services in ways that are appropriate to their needs and geography. Localities can be large or small depending on requirements. Within the present system it is difficult for a practice that is clustered with one neighbouring practice for fundholding management purposes to enter into an agreement with another neighbour that is not its fundholding partner.

### Successes so far

The list is longer than we expected at the outset. We have found that close working relationships have developed across the Consortium practices between both GPs and practice staff.

High calibre management has been very successful in attaining the targets set at the outset. (This quality of management skill would not be financially feasible for a single fund, as it would use up all of its management allowance.)

We have formed healthy purchasing alliances with our local providers and our Health Commission. These have allowed the introduction of two major services into our district. One (cardiology) is new to us, having been previously supplied from another Health District. We now have a visiting consultant who is based in the local District General Hospital. Access times have also been reduced by using a different provider, from six months in 1993, to six weeks in 1995 for an out-patient appointment and from 18 months to two months for an in-patient episode. The other service strengthens one that previously was perceived as weak. The improvements are available to the whole district and can be accessed equally by non-fund-holders.

We are building relationships with patient support groups and the local Community Health Council that we think will improve our ability to purchase care in a manner appropriate to their needs. The day-to-day contact GPs have with their patients means that they are likely to see most patients attending the secondary care sector on a fairly regular basis. As a matter of course the success or failure of a procedure or contact will be discussed. This is the basis of the success of fundholding and means that the advocacy role of GPs remains fundamental to its continuance. Whether it is necessary or appropriate to formalize this relationship further must be questioned, as the cost of widening the consultative process becomes substantial very rapidly. Only if the information gained by wider consultation is significantly different from that supplied by GPs would the extra cost and effort of obtaining it appear to be justified.

Joint purchasing with our Health Commission is developing, with joint discussion groups helping to formulate policy in many areas. The local Social Services Department is closely involved, and members of the Consortium board sit on joint Social Services/Health Commission consultative groups.

Liaison with the local Health Commission's Department of Public Health has been very productive and their support has been an invaluable source of advice on how to assess the health needs of the population.

## Where are we now?

The Consortium has shown itself to have many advantages over conventional 'stand alone' fundholding. Common aims mean greater purchasing power and closer working links are possible between the various member fundholders, especially in purchasing. These are often made more readily than between 'stand-alone' fundholders as there is an underlying mood of co-operation rather than competition. Diversity too can flourish within Consortia. All that is needed is a willingness by all members to be tolerant of the wishes of other practices, and to discuss potential developments with those likely to be affected.

There is no doubt that the large purchasing budget also gives more power to a Consortium to force changes on provider units. This can work to enable provider units to introduce changes, allowing them to encourage the more conservative consultants into changing their working practices.

There is an increased awareness of the need for fundholders to be responsible purchasers, and not to destabilize a provider or another fundholder unnecessarily. A Consortium can offer fundholders the ability to protect services that could be threatened by the careless or selfish purchasing of others, and better management is possible, resulting in more power to effect change and manage the fund efficiently. This management is enhanced by the need for GPs to discuss and agree purchasing decisions within the Consortium, leading to more informed contracting, with decisions being taken to benefit the widest possible population.

The regular meetings of the Consortium members offer a forum for the exchange of views on many issues, but especially those of service quality. The knowledge of member practitioners is effectively pooled and a greater understanding of the effectiveness of the secondary care sector develops. This in turn informs our contracting and will lead in time to a better service from our providers.

## Developing relationships

Figure 2 shows how we relate to other organizations. Purchasing is a responsibility that demands much of its administrators. With the large amounts of money involved, proper systems of

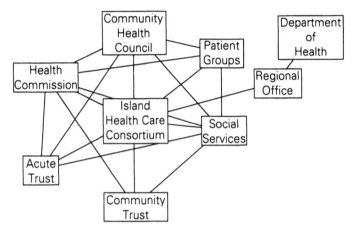

**Figure 2**  How do we relate to other organizations?

accountability have to be developed. For the foreseeable future
the NHSE regional offices will be retaining the role of supervising fundholding. However, much of the work will be carried
out by Health Commissions and the new integrated Health
Authorities after April 1996. As these Authorities are also
purchasers they have a responsibility to prevent a conflict of
interest arising between their purchasing role, their budget
setting and their monitoring role. This will prove difficult for
many authorities as they have until now been part of the
command and control approach to managing the NHS. A
considerable culture shift will have to take place to allow
fundholding to develop an appropriate relationship with its
relevant Health Authorities.

## Health Commissions

Relating to Health Commissions and integrated purchasing
authorities is going to be one of the most difficult problems of
the next stage of the NHS reforms. The passing of the command and control ethos from the management of the NHS is

likely to prove difficult for many. Fundholders will increasingly have to take into account the wider purchasing needs of their local areas when taking decisions. The Fundholding Account-ability Framework[1] published by the Department of Health in April 1995 lays down guidelines for the monitoring of fund-holding. These will need to be interpreted by both parties in a manner that recognizes the maturity of fundholding if prob-lems are to be avoided.

## Trusts

Most fundholders have at least reasonable working relation-ships with local NHS Trusts. It is often the clinicians within Trusts who, having lost some of their power as a result of the rise of fundholding, are the most reluctant to embrace new methods of working. Where they have been involved construc-tively by the purchasers, early in the contracting process, the result seems to be more acceptable to all. We also have a role in encouraging service developments in the Trusts within the finances available to us as purchasers.

## Local Authorities

Locally we are working with social services in a variety of groups, both directly and via joint policy groups organized by the Health Commission. There is GP purchaser representation on several joint commissioning advisory groups covering client groups, such as:

- children
- elderly
- mental illness
- learning difficulties
- drugs and alcohol problems.

It is increasingly necessary to maintain contacts with the Social Services Department as they control the discharge of many patients into the community, and problems in this area will simply delay discharge and block acute hospital beds.

## The health of the nation

As responsible purchasers, fundholders have to show where they are taking into account relevant *Health of the nation* targets[2]. Two targets are especially relevant to the Isle of Wight. We have been active in trying to reduce heart disease rates locally by introducing a cardiology service to the district. Additionally we have been working with the Health Commissions to achieve a comprehensive mental health service for local residents. We hope, that by improving these facilities, there will be a reduction in rates of death from ischaemic heart disease and better treatment of attempted suicide. These are the two most pressing problems on the Island from the *Health of the nation* targets.

# Where do we want to be?

We feel that there is still a need for further changes in the regulations governing fundholding. Becoming a fundholder, especially within the framework of a Consortium, should be easier with recognition of the mutual support function that arises from the co-operative approach. This can only come about with the support of the Department of Health and although there are some signs of support for such changes, there are, as yet, no specific proposals.

The changes in the regulations announced in the autumn of 1994, with increased management allowances and the reduction in list sizes, will allow the restructuring of some clusters into individual funds[3]. If budgets are set in a reasonably equitable manner then each of these funds should be self-supporting. It may be helpful to seek longer periods of time than a year before expecting funds to be in financial balance, especially where the volumes of activity are small.

It would still be helpful to see some more developments in the structure of fundholding. In particular, I would want to recommend and endorse the recognition of Consortia as a useful extension of fundholding. In our view, it is essential and the right of a Consortium to hold contracts. This would simplify matters immensely. We do not think that this would reduce the power of GP-directed purchasing. We have found that all our member GPs are quite committed to practice-based contracting, and members find having to cluster with other practices restricting.

The recently announced reduction in the minimum list size necessary to become a standard fundholder to 5000 patients is to be welcomed. For practices in a Consortium where mutual support is available, and some contingency management system could be operated, this limit could be further reduced.

Consortia are capable of covering overspends in funds where they occur by spreading the burden over a much wider patient base. This reduces the inequitable situation that occurs when an overspend by one member of a cluster has to be financed by the partner practice. Very different pressures apply within different practices, often arising from the varying styles of care provision that are practised and differing local requirements. These can be reflected in apparently widely different needs being found in apparently similar practices. Patient choice exerted over the years can produce a movement of patients. Those with higher levels of dependency may register with practices that have a caring reputation. Other patients who simply want quick access to basic services may opt for an 'efficient' practice with no waits for an appointment, but with less desire to uncover unmet needs and to undertake preventive care.

In order that Consortia are able to carry out some of these functions there is a need to look at the structure of the fund. Current arrangements appear to prohibit the use of companies limited by guarantee following the bad press attached to some early fundholders. This is unfortunate, as this form of structure would seem ideal for a multi-fund or consortium. It allows the latter to hold bank accounts and property in its own name, without making individual GPs financially liable should there be a problem with its finances. By being limited by guarantee, it could be non-profit making, making it difficult for it to be a route for the misuse of taxpayers money.

## What will we be able to do?

We feel that by moving the purchasing decision-making into the primary care sector, nearer to the patient, fundholding is producing a fairer and more efficient use of resources. We aim to build on our success to date by consolidating the good local services, improving the less effective ones, and purchasing from specialist providers those services that cannot be efficiently and effectively provided locally. Above all, I hope that provision of service will move closer to the patient, with as much care being provided from within primary care as possible. This will only arise if the resources required to nurture and sustain these innovative services are made available.

## Acknowledgements

Thanks to David Crawley and Mark Denman-Johnson of the Island Health Care Consortium for their help in producing this chapter.

# References

1  National Health Service Executive (1995) EL (95)54. *An accountability framework for GP fundholding.* NHSE, London.

2  Department of Health (1992) *The health of the nation. A strategy for health in England. Appendices A and C.* HMSO, London.

3  National Health Service Executive (1994) EL (94)79. *Developing NHS purchasing and GP fundholding.* NHSE, London.

# The primary care agency  7

*Roger Edmonds and Robert Sloane*

## The context

With the introduction of the internal market, the new GP contract and the shift towards care in the community, the 1990s have introduced profound changes in the way the NHS is run. At the heart of the changes is a wider concept of citizenship informing the way society views public services. There is now an increasing expectation that those services should be organized to meet the specific needs and preferences of individuals. Inherent in this policy is greater local empowerment and less central prescription.

For the NHS, which has been a monopolistic organization, this represents a culture change of immense proportion. Although the NHS was never a truly national service in the strict corporate sense, it had, over the years, evolved a blueprinting behaviour. Central planning and policy, driven by norms and standards, were designed to influence service delivery down to the finest detail. RHAs brought a tight discipline to bear on the strategic planning process, resulting in a rationally planned model, balancing resources within an equity framework. In contrast, the vision of today's NHS is of a service which is not only more devolved but which also has an in-built flexibility to be responsive to different patterns of assessed health need. Free-market forces challenge the rational planning that preceded them. The emphasis now is on localities, the natural communities where people live, work and associate. Such communities are sometimes, but not always, neatly described by administrative boundaries.

In some respects the new outlook is reminiscent of the pre-1948 NHS era. Then there was, in many places, a sense of community and a desire for local self sufficiency, upon which were laid the foundations of today's NHS. Public libraries are rich with the history of voluntary subscription, benefaction, charitable donations and philanthropy which provided health services, mainly hospitals, for communities of all sizes. Frequently local GPs were commissioned as figureheads, leaders and advisers in the local fund-raising efforts. Health had a high profile and was a matter of civic interest. What could and could not be afforded was openly debated and hard decisions were taken. Although the present NHS was built on the old networks, during its early years, local communities lost their influence and in most cases their interest. Many would argue that the very creation of the NHS led to a dependency culture and an expectation that the state would, and should, provide.

The proud legacy of that early period remains very much in evidence today, and is characterized most frequently in market towns by the presence of cottage or community hospitals. Strong historic encirclements of active GPs supporting and working in these hospitals have since the 1990s been given a renewed stimulus and the opportunity to provide an alternative pattern of care to that of the District General Hospital. Good examples of this configuration are to be found all over the UK.

High levels of community engagement in the organization and delivery of health care have been, and still remain, a potent force. Given that one of the principal objectives of the *Working for patients* reforms[1] was to make more explicit the connection between health investment and health outcomes, a resurgence of public participation may well result. This is not solely about the ability of local communities to raise money, although that may prove to be a decisive factor in future levels of service, as pressure on the public purse intensifies.

While individuals have played a significant role in the changes, the climate following the major reforms has also had the dramatic result of enabling GPs to act with greater effect on behalf of their patients. As a microcosm of the wider contracting process, GP fundholding has clearly had spectacular results.

Entrepreneurial primary care behaviour moving in concert with the wishes of local people can radically improve patient care. Small, close knit communities seem ideal test beds for experimenting with new models of local relevance. New patterns of working from Rye in Kent[2] to Nairn in Scotland[3], tend to support this contention.

Recognizing this context, it is now possible for a community of 50–100 000 people found in such market towns as Andover with several fundholding practices and a community hospital, to join forces and produce an exciting new model for a Primary Care Agency. In such communities, a broad range of well-developed local services is often to be found, including acute, community and mental health services. In rare instances, these may be run as separate Trusts as in the case of Andover or, as is more frequently the case, under locality management arrangements as part of a larger NHS Trust.

In many respects, the idea of a Primary Care Agency is simply the next step along the continuum beyond total fundholding. It is a federation or co-operative of small health care businesses led by GPs, incorporating many Community Health Services. In Andover, these services are provided by a small local Trust formed in 1992, of which GPs were the keenest advocates. The model is characterized by:

- closer working, possibly integration between GP practices and the local hospital management

- delegated responsibility for primary care led purchasing of secondary care

- increasing healthy alliances particularly in health and social care
- continuing education in primary care
- greater involvement of the local community in health affairs.

# The rationale

The rationale for developing this new model in communities such as Andover is derived from the following ten themes.

## Primary care purpose

A common aim of small health care businesses is to develop the scope of primary care and provide as many services in or close to patients' homes as possible. Moving the provision of services closer to the daily lives of patients is now increasingly possible because the range of services which can be provided outside hospitals has increased, as a result of technological changes in patient care, and the uprating of the skills of the primary care team. This orientation helps to reinforce the primacy of the voluntary and informal relationship between GP and patient. It also bestows on the GP greater gate-keeper control over the remainder of the health care system which is designed to provide a support service to the GP. Under this model, greater emphasis can be placed on primary and community care, admissions to hospital becoming less frequent and only for more highly specialized care.

## Contracting

In order for the Agency to deliver its primary care objective, funding also needs to be close to the patients. The Andover

Primary Care Agency looks to be funded on a locality basis, bringing together GMS and per capita based HCHS funding, with two principal financial duties:

1  acting as purchaser to subcontract for secondary care and specialist services from neighbouring Acute Trusts

2  acting as provider to manage direct support to primary care teams, to include health visiting and district nursing and ultimately a full range of hospital and community care.

Contracts will be structured in order to place the 'ownership' of patients firmly with GPs, their pathway into more technical levels of care being reported back to and validated by GPs. Furthermore, imaginative management of the contracting process may stimulate competition among providers based in District General Hospitals, resulting in a more detailed review of service performance. Willing support from Health Authorities, keen to develop locality purchasing is a key prerequisite for success here.

## Value for money

One of the political sensitivities flowing from the reforms has been the increased transaction costs and the apparent spawning of bureaucrats, particularly in the areas of accounting and information technology. Debate will continue to rage as to whether the service is over- or under-managed, but undoubtedly attention will remain on management costs. For local small health care businesses to co-operate and create a management service bureau, an agency arrangement is highly advantageous, particularly if the resultant savings can be redeployed into direct patient care. A federation or co-operative of fundholding practices can now use the opportunities of funding envisaged by EL(94)79[4] to generate considerable funds for the management of their services, both in terms of assessing the health needs of their patients, administrative costs and contractual arrangements with local providers of all kinds. Management costs can (and this may well prove to be of vital importance in the years to come) be reduced by sharing and delegating management processes across all the fundholders and the local hospital.

## Information

The NHS information management and technology (IMT) strategy places a premium on secure, confidential person-based information which, through integrated systems, will be shared across the NHS. The realization of that goal is still some way distant with artificial organizational boundaries and technical barriers preventing the smooth exchange of common information. Not only is this clinically and managerially inefficient, but more importantly it presents a bewildering discontinuity of information to patients using the service.

The IMT infrastructure depends on ensuring that there is adherence to standards which will then allow parts of the NHS to start making the connections which lead to better information flows to support the contracting process. In a locality context like Andover where there is a strong sense of common purpose and where the variables are fewer, the chance of a successful implementation of the strategy is greatly enhanced. Further, the Andover Agency will be ideally placed to fulfil the function of epidemiological mapping to inform health needs analysis, health promotion and clinical audit. It seems axiomatic that this work is undertaken where the information is, where it is best understood and where there is a clear incentive to collect it. The power of GP databases is yet to be fully unlocked, but within the Agency model the potential exists to assemble this on a locality basis and overlay it with information from other organizations, notably Social Services and the voluntary sector.

## Social care

That health and social care have remained organizationally separated for so long has been one of the greatest obstacles to the integration, and continuity of care for individuals. People receiving care are only interested in whether or not their care is co-ordinated, coherent and that it works for them. Collaboration at field worker level can be exceedingly good, but more often despite the system rather than because of it.

Early signs from the UK suggest that locality purchasing and contracting can bring health and social services together. Local Primary Care Agencies will be in a strong position to attract, and contract for, services from a multiplicity of providers, and social care should logically be part of this network.

## Education

GPs have always prided themselves on being able to meet new crises and stresses as they arise. Changes in information technology, management processes, and new purchasing requirements are contemporary examples of the need for further adaptation.

Evidence from existing purchasing projects suggests that for a locality purchasing group to operate successfully the following activities in particular may need enhancement[5].

- The ability to make locality purchasing sensitive to local needs, but in a situation of actual or potentially reduced resources, indicates that negotiating skills will need to be highly refined and flexible.

- The networking of clinicians, both medical and non-medical, is highly desirable, highlighting the ability of nurses, health visitors and other professionals to garner evidence about patients' needs, both real and perceived.

- The drawing up and use of realistic treatment and referral protocols will pay dividends in terms of the effective use of resources, and requires consultation with several key groups of clinicians, including GPs, practice nurses and providers including hospital consultants and managers.

- PHCT representatives and leaders will need to be credible and influential and their workload will need generous support.

- Postgraduate education and continuous professional development needs to take account of the new stresses and educational needs of all the members of the PHCT. Locality based, multidisciplinary education should be encouraged, and the teaching should be learner centred and of high quality.

## Independent and voluntary sector

No chapter about the future would be complete without reference to the independent sector. Politically, there appears to be a continuing commitment to a publicly funded NHS but, that means of delivery may well entail a kaleidoscope of providers, including a growing involvement of the independent sector. The policy is to be welcomed where it brings additional investments into the NHS, shares risk and for small organizations enables developments that would otherwise be unaffordable. On this basis the idea of a 'private' Primary Care Agency would sound fanciful. However, the notion of an Agency which contracts, through joint ventures, services in psychiatry, pathology, personnel management and plumbing, does not.

The Agency must also be in a position to harness and support the wide-ranging contributions of the voluntary sector. Informal networks, so powerful in the smaller community, can augment the more formal linkages that seem to pivot on joint planning arrangements.

## Public participation

Citizens are already being encouraged to take greater responsibility for their own health affairs and in the running of an organization which they pay for. Their opinions are increasingly sought in determining local health priorities and formulating matters of policy. Yet they are rarely involved to the same degree as in the period predating the NHS. Arguably, in smaller communities, people have been able more consistently to demonstrate their loyalty to a much loved local hospital, particularly if it comes under threat.

This degree of civic interest and sense of community identity should form the basis of true needs-led locality purchasing. By their very nature, communities will differ and investment patterns should reflect this.

Within the ever tightening fiscal climate there will still be room for voluntary support and fund-raising effort. This is a strength within any organization and one that is to be encouraged.

Perhaps less heralded is the seam of professional skills and capabilities which can be drawn upon to aid the management of health care. Good chairmen and non-executive directors in the reformed NHS have made outstanding contributions through the application of their commercial and professional experience. Whether in an appointed or elected mode, local people of this standing can certainly add management capacity in a voluntary or remunerated role.

To tie in to the local community, the Primary Care Agency will use a variety of different media to communicate with the public, including information giving points, the news media and public service networks.

## Outcome and audit

It is of vital importance that the Primary Care Agency ensures that its activities are of the highest possible quality, with management and clinical processes which are scrutinized and exposed to audit and outcome measures. This implies defining at an early stage, a series of standards by which management and clinical performance can be measured. The patient, as consumer, must and ought to have a vital role in this process. Essential qualities for the organization to be able to succeed and grow harmoniously within the community are:

- good communications and good accessibility, to stimulate and enhance the free flow of information, with suggestions and complaints that are dealt with effectively and are seen to be so

- good and effective housekeeping in the organization

- staff who know how to listen and act on what they hear.

As far as clinical issues and activities are concerned, we have found in Andover that there is a need for close co-ordination with the Medical Adviser to the local Health Commission who plays a vital role in advising about the impact of new therapies and remedies, and of the significance of national and local guidelines. The Agency's Medical Advisory Committee must stimulate consultation with local clinicians in order to draw up guidelines and protocols on such topics as prescribing and referral activities which are objective, robust, acceptable and measurable.

A Primary Care Agency should be able to take the lead in drawing up a framework of local outcome measurements and in grasping the nettle of such contentious but vital issues as value for money and clinical effectiveness. A consortium of doctors who have sufficient ambition and drive to have set up the Agency, will already have crossed the threshold of successful discussions and negotiations among themselves to manage these problems.

## Medical advice

The dilemmas which are thrown up by setting the health needs of the individual against the health gains for the community, can be nowhere more acute than in the situation where the doctor is responsible for deciding whether funds are available to pay for remedies that the patient needs.

The executives of future Primary Care Agencies will have responsibility for several million pounds, and therefore must be able to draw upon robust and timely advice concerning the most effective ways of using resources. This advice will need to be drawn from a widespread network of carers of all description, and we see the ultimate executive body as a small group of GPs from all the surrounding practices, with standing nursing and managerial input. This body will need to meet regularly and the time they spend will need to be protected, and should not be an addition to their normal work-load. As acceptable representatives they will have demonstrated qualities as doctors and leaders which are well above average commitment. Generous locum payments will therefore be necessary.

## Future development

Undoubtedly, the idea of a Primary Care Agency will be of great relevance in small and medium sized communities. Each of the communities will differ in how much of the infrastructure is already in place. Motivation for further change may be prompted either by missionary zeal or adversity. A common desire will be to retain (or gain) local influence in the policy making and resource allocation processes, to benefit patient care. The starting point may vary, but the developmental progression would seem to turn on the following key stages.

- Stage 1: Development of fundholding among local practices. All GPs in full communication with each other. Coordinated purchasing decisions. Good local hospital and community services.

- Stage 2: Total fundholding well rooted. Per capita funding flowing into the community. Needs-assessed locality purchasing well established. GPs acting as advisors to providing organizations.

- Stage 3: Structural change. Fundholding and Trust organization (whole or part) translated into a new structure. GPs with Board level positions controlling local hospital and community services, but also contracting in secondary care.

In full maturity, we expect that a local Primary Care Agency in Andover will probably require a new formal organization into which GP fundholding and NHS Trust services are both subsumed. This new model will vary in scope and size depending on the scale of community to be served. That this new organization will have both purchasing and providing roles should not be regarded as an obstacle, as the dual remit is currently undertaken by GP fundholders and a good many NHS Trusts. There will, however, be questions of probity, corporate governance and contestability which will need to be addressed.

For those contemplating the future beyond total fundholding, the Primary Care Agency has a logical appeal, by undertaking all of the purchasing and most of the providing in a community setting.

## References

1  Department of Health (1989) *Working for patients.* HMSO, London, p 3.

2  Millar B (1992) We can work it out. *Health Service J.* **102**: 13.

3  Tucker H (1994) *Nairn pilot site report and locality plan.* Scottish Office, Edinburgh.

4  National Health Service Executive (1994) EL (94) 79. *Developing NHS purchasing and GP fundholding.* NHSE, London.

5  Report to Chelsea and Westminster Commissioning Agency (1994) Office for Public Management; para 15 (v).

# The city multi-fund: a mechanism for primary care locality development

**8**

*David Paynton*

The East Southampton Multi-fund is a local association of fundholding GP practices which came together in 1994 as a co-operative group. A proportion of the management allowance is pooled collectively in order to form a strong purchasing team, acting on behalf of the practices. The Multi-fund, representing over 60% of the population in a defined geographical area, has major implications for health care for the whole area. The Multi-fund allows practices to develop their rich potential purchasing power to provide a framework, not only for the purchasing of secondary services, but also as an engine driving forward primary care development. The Multi-fund sees itself influencing health care strategy beyond the boundaries currently covered within the strict remit of fundholding and developing a purchasing strategy on the basis that we only need to purchase from secondary care that which cannot be effectively provided in primary care. The Multi-fund, being an association of independent practices, can develop as a body while at the same time recognizing and respecting that a diversity of approach is part of the richness of general practice. Accordingly, it provides a structure for both contemporary community organization and sustaining traditional smaller practices.

# Historical perspective

The Multi-fund evolved from a local purchasing Consortium established soon after the 1992 general election. Starting its life as a loose structure involving fundholders and non-fundholders it tried to address some local issues in an attempt to influence the purchasing strategy of the Health Commission and local providers. The purchasing Consortium itself saw its remit as covering the whole spectrum of health care, including acute services, maternity and links with social care. One of its earliest objectives was to develop community services including outreach clinics, the enhancement of community nursing and practice-based services such as physiotherapy.

Like any loose relationship there comes a time when it either has to evolve into something more formal or cease to exist. The decision to move down the Multi-fund route was influenced by a number of factors.

- Funding (including that for a project manager which had allowed it to develop) was coming to an end with no promise of continuation.

- A clear recognition that despite the rhetoric, GPs would only have a major influence on secondary care if they held the budget.

- Despite the fact that care was shifting into the community with increasing work-loads for GPs, there was no corresponding shift in financial resources.

- A recognition that the GP's voice was fragmented into a cacophony of competing sounds, diluting its effect, allowing powerful providers to drive forward their own agenda.

- In grouping together as a Multi-fund we could reduce some of the work-load as well as ensuring that we could afford a high calibre business manager to negotiate contracts on our behalf.

- The Purchasing Strategy of the Health Commission was too broad-based to focus on local needs, local issues or local development.

- In such areas as community nursing and mental health it was important to establish an overall local purchasing strategy shared by all fundholding practices, if care in the community was not to fragment.

- Many GPs had reservations about the potential for fund-holding to create a two-tier services, either between com-peting fundholders or between fundholders and non-fundholders and the Multi-fund option would min-imize the risk that this would develop within the locality.

- With four existing fundholding practices within the locality there was a general feeling that one by one we would eventually be forced down this route and in the last analysis it was preferable to make a collective decision.

- In a rapidly changing society, mirrored by changes in the health service, practices could simply not afford to shut their eyes to change if they were to survive.

- At the time of decision (November 1994) with a potential general election and change of government due within the next 3 years, the Multi-fund represented a structure which could evolve whatever the political future.

# Geography

The Southampton East Multi-fund covers a well-defined geo-graphical area bordered by two rivers, Southampton Water and a green belt area to the north. Two-thirds of the popula-tion live within the Southampton City boundaries, repre-senting a mainly working class area with three major council estates and mixed housing in between. A third of the population lives within the southern parishes of Eastleigh Council, being dominated mainly by an upwardly mobile population living in new estates which sprang up in the 1970s and 1980s. The population itself has a few black spots of deprivation but otherwise is fairly stable with a reasonable level of employment in traditional industries, such as the local shipyards, docks, British Aerospace and motor manufacturing. The overall population is approximately 120 000 people and the Multi-fund comprises 12 practices forming 10 fundholding units covering 75 000 patients.

Health care is influenced by a strong hospital dependency culture created by the local University Hospital. Like many large University Hospitals the culture within is strongly influenced by the needs of the institution rather than necessarily looking to the needs of the community. Where strong community services have developed within the district it has usually been in rural areas such as the New Forest with a community hospital as a base. It is in these rural areas where traditionally primary care has been strongest. In Southampton East, like other urban conurbations, there is a high degree of health and social morbidity impacting on primary care. GPs feel overwhelmed by day-to-day clinical demands. There is also a perception that yet again the inverse law applies with resources and community facilities moving away from the city, where arguably the need is greater, towards the more peripheral parts of the district. This has had an effect on GP morale, practice organization and at a time when entry into general practice is falling, substantial implications for recruitment.

## Organization

As in most cities, there is a mix of practices ranging from single-handed practices to large group practices. The 12 practices in the Multi-fund form 10 fundholding units. Eight units are represented by single practices with four smaller practices clustering together to form two units. There are four other existing fundholding practices and three non-fundholding practices still in the area. The Multi-fund's remit is that of a purchasing organization and each fundholding unit could fundhold in its own right. The structure and constitution of the Multi-fund sees the focus of control and responsibility still resting with each unit. Strategic decisions, therefore, by the Multifund can only be made if there is a clear consensus. The management allowances are channelled initially to the fund-holding unit with a proportion subsequently directed to a central account which funds the steering group, the business manager and his team and the negotiating and contracting process. The constitution currently being drawn up, with the help of the Isle of Wight Consortium, establishes a voting structure of the main management board with one vote per unit which is independent of that unit's list size.

There is an inner steering group consisting of four GPs, a practice manager and the project manager (eventually to be replaced by the business manager). The steering group meets monthly and the main business meeting bi-monthly. Minutes and agenda of the main business meeting are circulated to existing fundholders and non-fundholders within the locality. They are permitted to attend the main business meeting on the understanding that they may be asked to leave if there are confidential issues to be discussed and that they have no voting rights.

In addition to the main business meeting there is a practice managers' forum to provide mutual support recognizing that practice managers have a key role in the success of the Multi-fund. The practice managers' forum elects one of their members to sit on the steering group. The constitution allows practices, having given due notice, to opt out if they wish, which ensures that the organization itself recognizes the need to ensure that all practices involved have a degree of ownership of the decision-making process.

# Information technology

Early in 1995, computer consultants were appointed to oversee an IT strategy with the purpose of purchasing a unitary fund-holding system for the Multi-fund. Many practices hoped to develop their practice-based system on the back of a contract for the fundholding system. A unitary fundholding computer system leads to advantages by virtue of bulk purchasing as well as ensuring that data is processed uniformly, which enhances the purchasing and contracting process and negotiating position of the business manager.

Many practices' clinical systems are becoming obsolete in 1995 and if practices can purchase a new clinical system on top of the package by which the Multi-fund purchases the fundholding system, then this raises the exciting prospect of a common clinical system across the locality. This facilitates the process of identifying and collating the health needs of individual patients right across the locality and collating this information to develop a locality health plan, based on the unique data which is held by practices.

# Out-of-hours centre

Parallel to the development of the Multi-fund is the setting up of a locality out-of-hours assessment centre in a local branch surgery staffed on a co-operative basis according to list size. The centre is open at weekends and evenings up to midnight. The majority of the 13% of calls occurring between midnight and 7.00 am are provided by Healthcall, the commercial deputizing service. The out-of-hours centre's development has a number of implications for primary care and the Multi-fund.

- A recognition that out-of-hours demands have made the lives of GPs and their families intolerable, a factor which is affecting recruitment.

- An attempt to get to grips with the escalating out-of-hours demand, which inevitably occurs in a city population.

- A recognition that there is an increasing shift of chronically ill patients into the community, as a result of early discharge from hospital, day case surgery, changes in terminal care, community mental health and an increasing number of frail and elderly people in residential care. In urban areas this requires a development of a new medical primary care infrastructure to cover the out-of-hours period.

- The development of an overall strategy for health care out of hours which allows us to bring together other agencies, such as the district nursing service, social services, ambulance services and the Accident and Emergency Department whose function also impacts on out-of-hours primary care in the community.

- A change in the culture of expectation by encouraging patients to come to the centre unless their condition requires a home visit on medical grounds.

- The linking of the out-of-hours centre to individual practices' computer systems through connections already developed in the Multi-fund itself.

- The use of our potential purchasing power to negotiate a more equitable contract with Healthcall for cover in the night hours.

- Facilitating the process by which GPs from different practices get used to working with each other in an atmosphere of mutual trust at an operational level.

## Developments

In 1995, the development of the locality Multi-fund is still at an early stage. Many, both inside and outside the group, had reservations that GPs, who by their nature have to have a thick skin to survive, would not be able to work together. The Multi-fund, however, has created a model by which practices in stressed urban areas can group together in a mutual partnership, both as a purchasing organization and as a way of enhancing their provider role. As a result, the East Southampton model has a number of advantages.

- It allows practices and GPs to involve themselves as much or as little as they wish in terms of purchasing secondary care services.

- It allows us to develop a common training package which brings together GPs and practice managers in order to provide mutual support.

- GPs with an interest in a specific area are able to develop and influence the overall purchasing strategy which gives them increased job satisfaction as well as mutually benefitting the Multi-fund as a whole.

- The Multi-fund is able to build a picture of the overall needs of the community and develop a locality health plan which it can share with the local Department of Public Health. For this locality plan to have relevance effective links must be made with other agencies such as the City Council, Community Health Council, Social Services and Housing Departments.

- With the increasing shift of care into the community the Multi-fund (and the out-of-hours centre) allows us to develop a community framework for health care.

- The Multi-fund allows us to negotiate with powerful providers on an equal footing in order to encourage the development of locality services such as physiotherapy, ultrasound and outreach clinics which have previously been blocked.

- The model not only allows us to purchase secondary care from service providers, but also to purchase specific services from each other if an individual has a specific expertize, such as an interest in endoscopy, acupuncture or minor surgery.

• The organizational framework allows GPs to develop a parallel career for themselves while at the same time benefitting local health care. The Multi-fund also provides an umbrella allowing smaller practices which still offer a good personal pastoral service to maintain their development.

## The future

At present, in 1995/6, the Multi-fund remains a simple co-operative purchasing organization. Where is has developed a provider role, as in the out-of-hours service, it is still doing so on a co-operative basis. Clearly there is a potential to develop a degree of mutual trading between the respective practices but it is still too early to say whether the Multi-fund as an organization will confine itself to the contracting process or start to employ health care providers directly on its behalf. This will depend on future political developments and on decisions on whether fundholding is extended to include acute, maternity and/or social care.

GPs, despite their heavy clinical work-load, now have a unique opportunity to influence decision-making directly. In responding to this challenge, together with the challenges of fundholding, they have to move from being a reactive cottage industry to think in terms of forward planning, investment in the future, business and health plans. This will have a major impact on primary care development which will allow a mechanism by which health care resources can flow into primary care and ensure that secondary care purchasing is driven by the needs of primary care, rather than the converse, which has been true until now.

## Acknowledgements

With grateful thanks to Jean Roberts-Jones, our project manager, without whom the Multi-fund or the out-of-hours service would not have got off the ground.

# The integrated community care practice: general practice, citizenship and community care

**9**

*Patrick Pietroni*

The current dilemma facing general practice is whether, under the pressure of the 1990 reforms, it will retreat back into a set of core competencies which reflect its attachment and dependency on the medical model or whether it will embrace the responsibility of total care. If it accepts the latter, it will need to transform itself into the discipline of community care.

Sir Geoffrey Vickers, writing about community medicine, or the 'world of the well' as he called it, emphasized the need for the concepts of personal doctoring (general practice) and social medicine (public health) to come together to enable the new field of community care to flourish. Like many pioneers he was ahead of his time and few of his writings are well known within general practice. Nevertheless, he helped to identify a future direction for general practice which is even more relevant today than when he wrote in the 1970s. In describing his vision of community medicine he wrote:

> 'It is responsible for managing in the world of the well, the human estate of sickness and mortality. I include in this the management of the non-pathological crises of life, birth, growth, senescence, death – and the management of illness whether curable or not. I include the relief of suffering and in living with disability, whether

transient or permanent. Limitation of disturbance in all the social systems which an illness disturbs, notably, the household in which it is to be contained and partnership with the layman or more often lay woman who is primarily charged with the care of the sick individual, in the community and chiefly stressed by that responsibility'[1].

## Need for a vision

I believe Sir Geoffrey Vickers provides us with a vision which serves both the individual need and the community in which that individual resides. Before exploring it in detail, it is helpful to remember that the developments in general practice since the inception of the NHS have been characterized by certain phases, some propelled by need, some by a 'call to arms', some by visionary appeal and some by collective effort. These phases have included:

- the escape from hospital medicine
- the establishment of a separate clinical discipline
- the influence of Michael Balint and others on the consultation
- the drive for educational expertise
- the collection of data and clinical audit
- the move towards practice teams
- the emphasis on health promotion
- attempts at managerial proficiency
- current developments in fundholding and primary care led purchasing.

At the centre of these changes has been the consistent belief that the unit of general practice still remained that moment when, in the intimacy of the consulting room, one human being in distress confides in another human being whom he trusts. It is this focus on personal care that has epitomized British general practice and which in survey after survey patients report they value most in their GP. Some of the phases outlined above have challenged this tenet and some have attempted to strengthen it. It has become increasingly clear that to offer personal doctoring without reference to the context in which it is delivered (the patient's family, the practice team, the community needs, and the financial implications) is counter-productive. Similarly, to provide an impersonal set of health or social care packages, which are determined largely by their unit cost, will lead to a system of care which repels most professional groups and devalues that which is most valued. Unfortunately, the response by the professional bodies to the 1990 reforms has been dominated by their sense of loss of their professional freedom and autonomy. There has been little attempt to grapple with the changing nature of professional practice[2] or the crisis of professional knowledge[3]; thus the responses have appeared largely defensive.

Again, Sir Geoffrey provides a far more balanced critique and illustrates how appreciative behaviour (values, ethics, moral judgements), are central to any debate regarding market forces. Vickers argued persuasively that one cannot use the market as a regulator in matters affecting life and death. 'A resource that is inexpansible, indispensable and over-scarce, can no more be distributed through the machinery of the market than can the places in too few lifeboats on a sinking ship'[4]. Such issues must rest on the deliberate exercise of human judgement, and the exercise of what Vickers called 'balancing through time a host of disparate criteria, not all of which, usually not one of which, can be fully satisfied'. The tendency for Western societies to believe that automatic regulators can substitute for deliberate human regulation based on ethical principles derived largely, Vickers believed, from a change in what he called the appreciative setting associated with the Enlightenment. It lay at the heart of what he held to be the weakness of Western culture. This weakness can be best exemplified by the contrasting notions of the autonomous individual and the responsible person, and is central to the debate regarding direction for general practice.

## Citizenship and the patient

The comparatively recent introduction of the computer has enabled us to describe patients by age, sex and occupation together with certain parameters linked to levels of demand (Jarman score). These have proved useful for much of the clinical and administrative work undertaken in general practice, but it leaves out one of the more important factors that determines health-seeking behaviour, 'health belief'. Within a small practice (approximately 5000–8000), it is possible, using a modification of Maslow's hierarchy of need[5], to identify three distinct groups of patients, each having different needs and different expectations for care. It is important to accept that someone in the third group will, on occasion, want to be treated as someone in the first group and vice versa. Increasingly health care delivery systems will need to reflect the pluralistic model of total care.

### Basic survivors
These are patients who are barely surviving, overburdened by family, financial and housing problems. Their demands may be couched in physical terms but their needs are often psychological, social and spiritual. They may form part of an ethnic minority group suffering prejudice and discrimination. They may be elderly, single, isolated, living out a social death often while waiting for the physical death that will release them from their suffering. They form a dependent relationship with their GP and look to him or her to provide a form of pastoral care which many GPs strive to meet.

## Conspicuous consumers

These are the users or customers of our service and will want the health centre to operate as an efficient one-stop supermarket store. They want easy access, Saturday morning surgeries, long opening hours, courteous attention, efficient administrative systems and a wide range of products on offer. They seek information, so as to get the best buy and are often influenced by fashion and the latest medical advance, such as annual cholesterol checks, osteopathy for back problems, regular 'flu jabs. They are keen to have choice and will be quick to complain about perceived deficiencies in the system.

## Self actualizers

These are our clients who wish to be given explanations and information. Their need is for meaning and relationship. They wish to be more involved in their health care and they accept more easily the psychological and spiritual base to their disease. Their focus is towards empowerment and fulfilment and, increasingly, they will want to be involved in the ethical and moral debates surrounding medical procedures (eg resource allocation, high-tech procedures, euthanasia).

# Implications for practice

Many of these concepts of community care have already been explored by workers in the field. A comparison of three very different examples (Peckham experiment, 1935–1950[6], Glyncorrwg Community Practice, 1966–1988[7], and the Marylebone Health Centre, 1986[8]) illustrate how similar some of the underlying principles are.

## Peckham experiment

The pilot phase of this extraordinary experiment began in 1926. By the time it closed, it was attracting over 10 000 visitors a year. Its founders, Dr George Scott Williamson and Dr Innes Pearse, were in great demand as speakers and lecturers all over the world. The hypothesis they tested was that 'health is more infectious than disease'. They believed that if they provided an environment where individuals could come and participate in healthy activities, during which time they could be provided with periodic health examination, including information on how to promote their health, their quality of life would improve. Initially the experiment began in a small health centre in south London. It operated as a form of club and 30 families came together to organize it. It rapidly outgrew its accommodation and a new purpose-built building (the pioneer health centre) was designed and built in 1935.

It was hoped that, with the onset of the NHS, some of the principles embodied by the Peckham experiment would be incorporated within the planning of the new health centres then due to be built. Neither the importance of design of building nor the participatory nature of the experiment and, more importantly, not even the focus on health was seen as important. The health centres built within the NHS were managed and organized by doctors. The service offered was a reactive disease-based model and the preventive and promotional focus was minimized. With the death of the pioneers of the Peckham experiment, much of the impetus for their method of work was lost and attempts to keep the model alive have proved difficult.

Vickers, in his article on community medicine, acknowledged that 'the rate of change of mental habits is reckoned in generations'. One GP whose mental habits were ahead of his generation and who pursued the ideas propounded by Vickers, Dr Julian Tudor-Hart, has recorded his own pioneering work in the medical literature[7].

## Glyncorrwg Community Practice

The community in Glyncorrwg, a village in South Wales, was very closely involved with the mining industry but suffered like many industrial communities through the loss of its main source of employment. In 1966, 92% of men aged 16–64 were fully employed, but by 1986 this figure had dropped to 48%. Dr Tudor-Hart has emphasized the importance of social organizational cohesion on the health of a community and has emphasized the need to foster a new kind of doctor to meet the needs of the next few decades. He draws attention to the importance of the family group and community involvement in helping to sustain the health of individuals and suggests that doctors need to move away from a reactive, individually based, clinically oriented practice of medicine to one which is proactive, family and community based and which accepts the social, cultural, economic and political factors that influence health and disease.

Like the pioneers at Peckham, Dr Tudor-Hart has highlighted the importance of architecture and the built environment. He describes the impact of a swimming pool on the health and well-being of his patients. Likewise Vickers held the view that 'the most enduring signature that a man can inscribe on the world is a building. The whole physical milieu is increasingly a human artefact, and this artefact is a commitment ever more permanent and ever more potent for multiple good or ill'. The importance of architecture on community care is no better illustrated than in the third experiment where Vickers' ideas are being explored.

## Marylebone Health Centre

The Marylebone Health Centre is an ordinary general practice offering a traditional orthodox medical service to over 5500 patients. It is situated in central London and in 1987 began to experiment with different models of delivering community care. These experiments included:

- the use of complementary therapies (eg osteopathy, massage, herbal medicine, homeopathy) available as appropriate to patients

- a counselling and psychotherapy unit enabling many of the emotional and psychological concerns of patients to be dealt with directly

- a social care unit with outreach workers ensuring that the more vulnerable members of the community (eg elderly, homeless, single parents) receive direct access to a range of services that impact directly on their level of well-being

- a health promotion and health education unit providing a range of self-care and self-help activities encouraging patients to learn about and take more control of their own health

- a patient participation programme, run and staffed by the patients themselves, ensuring that volunteer activities (eg befriending, practical support, creche, telephone advice service, practice newsletter) are available to the community living near the health centre.

The site of the health centre, in the crypt of a church, provides an architectural site which is not only beautiful and aesthetically pleasing, but symbolizes the holistic nature of the project, paying attention to the whole person, psychologically, spiritually and socially, not just to the physical aspects.

This experiment in delivering community care was accompanied by a rigorous research study, and within the first 3 years, it became apparent that outcome measures of prescribing, investigative procedures and referral to specialists were substantially different from other practices with similar populations.

Of all the experiments undertaken at the Marylebone Health Centre, the one addressing social care has been the most difficult and taken the longest to demonstrate results, but it will probably turn out to be the most important for general practice and community care. It will be far more important than the introduction of complementary medicine for which the Centre has become known. There are now a series of programmes in place mostly run by patients but co-ordinated by an outreach worker which include:

- transport service for patients and their relatives
- decorating and minor repair service
- befriending (sitting with elderly patients)
- telephone contact, once a month for all the over 75s
- single parent club
- newsletter, three times a year
- language interpreter service
- homeless accommodation service
- crisis listening service (drop-in)
- swimming club
- movement to music
- choir
- elderly–toddler afternoons
- yoga classes
- reminiscence group
- volunteer groups (helping with clerical and administrative work)
- informal complaints procedure (organized by a specialized group of parties)
- welfare rights clinic.

## Conclusions

Table 9.1 compares some of the principles that underpin these three experiments and points the way forward. For general

**Table 9.1** A comparison of the Peckham, Marylebone and Glyncorrwg experiments

| Peckham experiment | Marylebone Model | Glyncorrwg Community Practice |
|---|---|---|
| • Our concept is that health is a mutual synthesis of organism and environment. | • There is an inter-connectiveness between human beings and their environment. | • We must accept the full implications of both groups and individuals practising an open style of medicine. |
| • In this new field there was no existing knowledge of well-defined entities, relationships, dynamics and regularities which the bionomist might encounter. | • Tolerating uncertainty, taking risks and making mistakes are part of the stepping stones in the search for wholeness. | • We need to admit to ourselves, our colleagues and our patients what we do not yet know and what we have not yet done. |
| • Approaching conventionally as a scientist, how then is he to fulfil the technological requirements of assessment – how is he to measure his material? | • Research studies should pay due cognisance to the moral, ethical and financial consequences of their outcome. | • We must learn to apply scientific principles imaginatively to the health care of people as they live and work. |

**Table 9.1** *continued*

| Peckham experiment | Marylebone Model | Glyncorrwg Community Practice |
|---|---|---|
| | • This does not mean that we discard science, rather that we respond imaginatively, actively and creatively, as scientists to discover the construction of health and disease as a social process. | |
| • Is it essential to grasp the processes that sustain and develop an individual's health care other than the processes that underlie and govern his disease? | • Health and disease lie along a continuum and represent the organic-intrinsic state of harmony with the universe. | • We must learn to deal with measurable, continuously distributed variables in which disease (requiring active remedial intervention) is difficult or even impossible to separate from health (requiring active conservation). |

**Table 9.1** *continued*

| Peckham experiment | Marylebone Model | Glyncorrwg Community Practice |
|---|---|---|
| • Supper is an important time of meeting for all members of the staff. At times these lead to discussions that may run deep. | • It will not be possible for doctors to address the health problems of the twenty-first century unless we learn how to share our power, not only among our colleagues in the health team, but also with our patients. | • We must accept that effective medical care and, even more, the effective conservation of health requires an enormous range of skills other than those of doctors, including skills of other medical, nursing and health professionals who have been systematically subordinated to and exploited by us and our predecessors and that our own skills will survive only if they can be shown to be useful. |

**Table 9.1**  *continued*

| Peckham experiment | Marylebone Model | Glyncorrwg Community Practice |
|---|---|---|
| • Health of which we were in search, demanded that the family should shoulder the responsibility for its own actions – this was basic to the hypothesis on which the work was conceived. | • Users of health-care services need to be offered knowledge, skills and support to enable them to take an active interest in their health and emotional well-being. They can also share the responsibility for helping to maintain the organization designed to promote health and community care. | • We must accept patients as colleagues in a jointly designed and performed production in which they will nearly always have to do most of the work. We must look to a more dependable alliance with the ordinary people we serve. |

practice to transform itself to address the needs within the next decade some or all of the following need to occur.

- The willingness of the practice to broaden its definitions of health care, not in name only.

- The expansion of the primary health care team to include colleagues from social care and the development of a teamwork ethos which does not privilege one form of care, be it body (physical, mind, psychological), soul (spiritual) or environmental (social) over another.

- The designation of proactive care through outreach as being integral to the task of community care.

- The recruitment and active involvement of volunteers from the practice population and the encouragement and empowerment of all those active individuals to participate in the practice itself.

- The recognition of the informal carers present in each practice who have undertaken community care without support.

- The restructuring of the organizational base of general practice from a GP, partnership-based model to one which truly reflects the framework required for the delivery of an integrated community care practice.

None of these activities needs to interfere with the individual pastoral care that occurs when, in the intimacy of the consulting room, one human being in distress confides in another human being whom he trusts. This individual package of health care practice must always remain at the core of British general practice. However, to misquote Michael Balint, to meet the challenge of the future, general practice will need to pass through a 'limited though considerable change in its personality'[9].

# References

1 Vickers G (1984) Community medicine. In: Open Systems Group (eds.) *The Vickers papers*. Harper & Row, London.

2 Vickers G (1984) The changing nature of the professions. In: Open Systems Group (eds) *The Vickers papers*. Harper & Row, London.

3 Schön D (1992) The crisis of professional knowledge. *J Interprofessional Care*. **6**: 49–63.

4 Blunden M (1984) Geoffrey Vickers – An intellectual journey. In: Open Systems Group (eds.) *The Vickers papers*. Harper & Row, London.

5 Maslow A H (1954) *Motivation and personality*. Harper & Row, New York.

6 Pearse H I (1989) *The quality of life*. Scottish Academic Press, Edinburgh.

7 Tudor-Hart J (1988) *A new kind of doctor*. Merlin, London.

8 Pietroni P C (1995) *The Marylebone Experiment*. Churchill-Livingstone, London.

9 Balint M (1957) *The doctor, his patient and the illness*. Pitman, London.

# The GP based care network

## 10

*Tom Davies*

This chapter on organizational development in primary care is written in two parts. The first gives an outline sketch of the history of our general practice at Yaxley over the past 30 years, and how we have developed relationships within our primary health care team on the outskirts of Peterborough. The second part looks at the wider issues of communication between doctors and social workers, and why changes have not occurred as quickly as they might. I have avoided talking about structures because I believe that one should not impose one method of working on practices. Each should be helped to discover what works best for them, in their specific circumstances.

## Introduction

General practice has changed out of all recognition since 1950–1970, due to numerous factors. The formation of the Royal College of General Practitioners, in the face of much opposition, in 1952 started GPs thinking about issues of general practice at a time when most were still working single handed. The GP Charter of 1966 was central to helping GPs see the benefits of working together. Hasler notes that there was great ignorance at that time about doctors' knowledge of the function of health visitors, and ignorance about district nurse qualifications[1]. Changes that have had major implications on work-load for the primary care team over the past 25 years include:

- government reorganizations

- advances in technology

- consumerization with its increasing demands and expectations

- demographic shifts (there will be more than one million people in the UK over 85 years of age by 2001).

Change continues, and is a challenge. The present government's intention to make primary care drive the changes is to be welcomed, but there is concern at the speed of change. As people have moved from secondary to primary care, resources have not always moved, nor are appropriate arrangements put in place before the transfer of care.

The place of primary care as that which most patients choose to turn to for help continues to be well understood. Paradoxically, at a time when high technology medicine (eg near patient testing, the use of smart electrocardiograms and other technological monitoring devices) is moving increasingly into primary care, the social, psychological and spiritual needs of patients have never been more important for the primary health care team to consider. The advent of computerization has tremendous advantages in recording information that can easily be shared in an up-to-date format across the team, and increasingly between sites. However, use of IT imposes an extra initial work-load and a discipline on all the professionals using the technology that must be understood. The most important change required for successful implementation of community care is without doubt attitudinal not organizational.

# History of the Yaxley group practice

In 1959 ours was a two-man rural practice, with some 5500 patients. The two doctors covered their own on-call duties, and one wife worked as a dispenser. In 1964 the first nurse/receptionist was appointed and soon after a part-time secretary. Both appointments were very unusual at the time. A purpose-built surgery 'to last their lifetime' was opened in 1965, but by 1972/3 was already inadequate. In close collaboration with the local authority (pre-1974 reorganization) a purpose-built health centre was established and a third partner was appointed for the list size of 6200. A practice manager was recruited, along with a team of receptionists and two dispensers. The health centre was very well equipped with physiotherapy, chiropody and community dental suites. Even then the two senior partners had wished to build an adjacent six-bedded unit but this was turned down after appeal to the Secretary of State. At the same time a 20-bed hostel for disabled people was built on the same site and we have enjoyed the closest of working arrangements with the staff and residents ever since. Several outlying supported bungalows and houses now exist in the village and there have been very few problems. Staff attached to the health centre included a district nurse, two health visitors, a midwife and a school nurse. A psychologist spent a research year attached to the practice in 1977, looking at psychological problems and the effects of early intervention in general practice. Weekly welfare clinics were held in the large education room in the practice and continue to this day. A neighbouring single-handed GP retired soon after and this list was taken over by the junior partner in 1976.

I joined the practice in 1978, as a fourth partner in a practice of just over 8500 patients. I had been trained in London and had spent just two weeks in general practice as a student. I moved to Peterborough and joined the Vocational Training Scheme (VTS) which at that time was still voluntary. Here I met my future partner Ian Redhead who had established the VTS in 1973. While in my first training practice

I was attached to the local Social Services Department in Huntingdon in 1976 for two weeks. I have always been grateful for this early exposure to the work of social services. Much of what I saw opened my eyes and I hope it has helped in all relationships between social workers and myself since. My father, who was medically qualified, had been Director of Social Services of Liverpool since 1971, and so I had some knowledge of both sides of the equation.

The practice has been partially computerized since 1984 and fully computerized since 1989 when we put terminals on our desks. At present we have an 18-terminal computer system and hope to upgrade to a 26-workstation networked system in the summer of 1995. We bought the building from the DHA in 1988 and have extended it substantially since. We became a third-wave fundholding practice in 1993 and have moved physiotherapy back into the practice (it had moved in 1980 when open access physiotherapy was established). We dispense for some 5000 patients from the small outlying villages. We look after 60 pregnant women a year in our local General Practice Unit. At the present time, we have seven partners (six whole time equivalents) with 11 800 patients.

We hold twice weekly meetings. The Monday educational meetings are for all members of our primary health team. Business meetings occur on Fridays and are minuted. Minutes are sent to the staff, and the chairman of the Patients' Association. We have held regular inter-professional meetings for the past 10 years, and been away on working weekends to look at how the practice should develop. There are regular fortnightly staff educational meetings, and we close the surgery once a quarter for study afternoons.

The present attached staff include:

- district nurses
- school nurse
- speech therapist
- orthoptist

- community psychiatric nurse for the elderly
- health visitors
- physiotherapist
- chiropodist
- dietitian
- MacMillan nurse.

As a fundholding practice, most of these attachments were in place before 1993, but physiotherapy has moved back and the chiropody, orthoptic and dietetics services have been extended.

## Patients' Association

For over 20 years, the health centre has been the focus for provision of comprehensive community care in our Yaxley community, and provides a long standing, consistent place to obtain help. The strength of our liaison with the local community has undoubtedly been strengthened over recent years by the setting up of our Patients' Association in 1984. Most patients requiring information about services and help would probably turn to the Patients' Library first. The Patients' Association Committee meets monthly and has been responsible for providing much medical equipment through fund raising. Examples of the medical equipment purchased by the Patients' Association:

- chemical pathology machine
- respiratory monitoring (apnoea alarms)
- defibrillator
- nebulizers

- smart electrocardiogram
- overhead project and slide projector
- Resusci-Anni
- terminal care-two syringe drivers
- dinomapp self blood pressure monitor
- resuscitation equipment
- teletext modulator YAXFAX for waiting room
- ripple mattresses
- video-recorder
- skeleton.

The Committee provide leaflets and appointed a Patient's Librarian/Resources Officer in October 1991. This is partially funded by the Association and partially by the practice. In 1992 a club for the over 65s (the Age-well club) was started and their weekly social and educational meetings are held at the health centre on a Tuesday morning. The Association has been successful in maintaining a weekly dial-a-bus service that collects people without transport from outlying villages on Tuesdays.

The Practice Resource Officer, with a background as a legal secretary and in a Citizens Advice Bureau, is an obvious first contact for people with housing problems and for those wishing to find out more about Social Security claims. A newsletter is regularly produced, and several hundred leaflets are now available for patients. The library has over 600 books, and 20–30 videos and tapes, these are fully catalogued on a separate computer.

In April 1995 we started a joint patient/client held record project with the Social Services Department with a set-up grant from the local Health Commission.

# Hospital-at-home

We were one of the first three practices to pilot the concept of hospital-at-home in 1979. In the first phase, separate staff were employed but it soon came obvious that the scheme would be best placed within the control of the primary care team and in 1980 the scheme was relaunched in Peterborough with the District Nursing Sister being the key lead person. Nursing auxiliaries, after 4–6 weeks training, are with the patient up to 24 hours a day. The scheme has gone from success to success and the case mix includes patients who are terminally ill, seriously medically ill (strokes, heart attacks) and those discharged early from hospital (eg following a hysterectomy). The Peterborough early discharge for hip fractures has enabled the elderly to be successfully returned home sometimes as soon as the fourth or fifth post-operative day.

# Working with social workers

We have always worked closely with social services. We have regular interdisciplinary meetings, with our health visitors and district nurses being the key contacts for liaison.

For the past two years, we have had two social workers providing counselling sessions within the practice, and before that social workers regularly (weekly) held surgeries in our premises. We schedule our day so the partners meet before surgeries, and have 20 minute catch up periods in the middle of surgeries when over tea or coffee we catch up on our paperwork, and colleagues know they can catch any of us to discuss individual patients.

# Communication

Communication is the key, and we increasingly use our computer system as the up-to-date record. Attached staff are encouraged to use the computer system and record their contact with the patient. An essential way we share information is the 'Events book' kept on the back desk by the visits book where all important information is recorded. Emergency admissions, deaths, significant diagnoses are all recorded, and help, in a small community, to pass on essential information. Correct handling of terminal care and death is essential. To not acknowledge the death of a relative would not only be insensitive it would also seriously challenge the caring concept of primary care. Logging of all emergency admissions and thus informing colleagues who may be visiting at home again saves work and enables them to act appropriately (and visit hospital if appropriate). An increasingly important role we play is to help advise relatives about the care of their loved ones in hospital. In a practice of almost 12 000 patients, personal care may be difficult, but it is made possible by proper communication. The role of receptionists and others should not be forgotten. Knowledge of relationships and past events is significant and cannot be found in text books.

# Shared records

There has been much written about enabling patients, and helping them have information they (and their carers) need to take responsibility for themselves[2]. Several recent developments (eg the 'Caring for People' legislation, computerization of medical records, increasing mobility of patients and the increasing use of respite care), make the shared care of this group increasingly demanding. Problems seem to arise regularly because of the poor communications between the professionals involved. The development of the local GP Co-operative for out-of-hours visiting has raised questions about the problems doctors might have seeing patients with serious and complicated conditions without adequate information. There is undoubtedly an increase in morbidity in the community. Private residential homes now have clients who some 10 years ago would never have been allowed to leave hospital. As a practice we had often left the full records with some patients expecting to be seen in the next few days. To our knowledge no problems have arisen so far with such an arrangement. Patients have freely held their full Lloyd George medical records when moving around the Yaxley Health Centre. No problems have arisen on the occasions when they have chosen to have a peek!

A major problem for the PHCT is to know who else has contact with the patient. Use of the shared record, which is kept with the person or carer will enable up-to-date information to be accessed at the time the person is seen. A regular computer printout will be provided. The items contained on the printout are itemized in Table 10.1.

## GP based community care

There has always been an uneasy tension between doctors and social workers. Ian Gilchrist in 1979 documented some problems which may be relevant today for many practices[3]:

- inadequate provision of accommodation

- inadequate provision of telephone, secretarial help

- lack of discussion between social worker and seniors about aims of attachment

- lack of discussion between social worker and practice team about mutual hopes from the attachment

- absence of regular structured meetings

**Table 10.1**   Contents of shared record

Administration details

- Named GP
- Other named carers/agencies (with contact numbers)
- Hospital number and Consultant involved

Updated computerized encounter sheet

- Significant past history
- Repeat medication

Summary information

- Preventive medical data (eg blood pressure)
- Investigations
- Screening data (eg smears, mammography, cholesterol)

All appointments

Copies of important letters (including our referral letters –
proofs sent)

Copy of discharge letters (duplicate should already be given
to patients)

Other reports (eg optician's reports)

Self-help leaflets (eg asthma, diabetes)

- inadequate opportunities to discuss patients' problems
- absence of regular channels of communication with the
  practice

- no procedure for regular written communication about patient problems

- no channel of communication with senior staff to review the attachment

- inappropriate referrals

- professional groups using different language and lapsing into technical jargon

- personalities involved are incompatible.

Ignorance and suspicion about each other's roles still remain. There has not been clear understanding of each other's contribution. Undoubtedly all professionals are increasingly working under pressure, and adequate communications are often very unsatisfactory. No wonder the patients and clients have been confused. The stability of general practice and the fact that most GPs are in practice for many years provides consistency in long-term care. The frequency of contacts (most people still have an average of around four contacts a year each, which for a family of four may mean contacts every month) means that relationships can be built up over many years. Undoubtedly this is the great strength of general practice and the reason that GPs are responsible for most referrals to Social Services Departments.

# Workload of social workers in general practice

Gilchrist alo outlined the workload of attached social workers (Table 10.2)[3].

At Yaxley, much of the work that would elsewhere be done by an attached social worker is done by our Patients' Communications Officer. The attached social worker we had for two years did not see enough patients to justify appointments

**Table 10.2**    Workload of attached social workers

| | |
|---|---|
| Provision of appliances for the physically handicapped | 83.6% |
| Provision of services for the deaf | 35.2 |
| Provision of services for the blind | 55.3 |
| Advice about social benefits | 83.1 |
| Accommodation problems (rehousing) | 90.0 |
| Assisting client with problems arising from: | |
| •  Marital conflict | 87.7 |
| •  Marital separation | 80.4 |
| •  Contact with the law | 51.6 |
| •  Parental conflict | 75.8 |
| •  Others | 76.3 |
| Assisting with management of psychiatric illness | |
| •  Psychotic illnesses | 73.1 |
| •  Other psychiatric illness (depression, anxiety) | 84.0 |

continuing to be booked at the surgery. It may be that for some meetings the clients prefer the anonymity granted by seeing the social worker in a separate office, away from the practice. It is absolutely right that they have the choice.

# Hospital discharge

Discharge arrangements have seemed to be an arbitrary process in the past, delegated at short notice to junior medical staff, often just before the beds are required for the next patient. When patients are discharged to a new address it is still, in 1995, depressingly rare for arrangements to be made to obtain the services of a new GP until the patient is at a new home. Even then, the patient may be at the new home for a 'trial period' and not permanently register with the practice till the end of that time. Delays of up to three months are still not unusual before old records come through, and hospital correspondence may continue to be sent to the previous GP's surgery. People at a very vulnerable stage will be treated by professionals with inadequate knowledge.

## Ethical problems

Ethical problems should also be acknowledged, with the doctor often having more than one patient (carer and client) to look after. Potential conflicts over confidentiality, both within the family and with our social worker colleagues should be recognized, but with trust and a joint determination to work together these issues can largely be addressed. Personal attachments and relationships are the key. Patient-held records overcome the problems of professionals seeing the records as their responsibility alone.

## Definition of health and social care

Definitions of the differences between health and social care are arbitrary. Increasingly patients are confused by the fact that the NHS is free at the point of contact although charges may be levied for care arranged through the Social Services Department. In our practice the home care assistants often have many skills and experience, and the move to encourage the development of generic workers able to do simple health tasks (eg cutting nails, supervising medication) is enormously helpful and reduces the risk of several people being involved, which is an expensive use of professional time and bewildering for the client. The concept of one-stop care, where people can get the help they need in one setting is becoming popular, and to run social services in isolation from this is, I believe, unhelpful. The problems of non-congruous boundaries is still a major one, with health, housing and social services still often covering different areas.

## Care managers

Under the 'Caring for people' legislation, care managers are the lead people obliged to arrange packages of care for their clients. Liaison between the primary care team and care managers is essential. All should be known, and full details kept in the primary care record. Computerization will, I believe, help enable the proper sharing of information.

## Computerization

Over 80% of GPs keep computerized records with many using them on their desk tops for clinical recording. Many practices, such as our own, wish their attached staff to enter their encounters on the computer as well, and thus help inform everyone of their involvement. It is estimated that up to 10% of computerized practices have already abandoned the written record. Communications between GPs and hospitals, and soon between each general practice will enable information about patients to arrive more quickly and more accurately. Using the Read classification of patient data there should be standard codes by which information is exchanged, and nationally work is now underway looking at the terms that nurses, PAMs (Professions Allied to Medicine) and social workers use.

The modern GP computer system should enable each professional to have access to the information they need, and for it to be flexibly printed out. Too much time is wasted recording information twice, three times or even more. Patients already think that this information is freely transferred and are surprised and even annoyed when they realize the delays that exist in the present system.

## Conclusion

This has been a personal account of how a semi-rural 12 000 person practice has developed. The new NHS reforms have clearly had a major impact on the NHS but I believe the way forward still remains one of looking at attitudes of minds, and trying to change those, rather than tinkering with the structures of the organizations. Above all, the continuing development of general practice as the focus for one-stop care as a central point in the local community networks, depends on better communications between all those involved. From the historical perspective I believe we are now at the stage in the development of general practice where technology provides a window of opportunity for the sharing of information, to achieve this long sought after goal.

## References

1   Hasler J (1992) The primary health care team: history and contractual forces. *BMJ.* **305**: 232–4.

2   McLaren P (1991) The right to know. *BMJ.* **303**: 937–8.

3   Gilchrist I, Gough J B *et al.* (1978) Social work in general practice. *J. Coll General Practitioners.* **28**: 675–86.

# The Primary Care Trust: co-ordination for cohesion

# 11

*Nigel Starey*

Primary care is defined in a variety of ways, but for the purposes of this chapter I shall restrict it to first contact, continuous, comprehensive and co-ordinated care provided to an undifferentiated but registered population. While international comparisons show that the management and co-ordination of primary care models vary, they do provide support for the concept of primary care as the foundation of an efficient health service[1]. In the UK, the link between clinical management by an individual's registered personal physician and the rest of the NHS needs examination in the light of changes in society and changes in medical practice. There are dangers in relying too heavily on competition as a lever for change, as it may promote further perverse or inappropriate incentives rather than develop effective care. Nor should fundholding be regarded as a sound link until it operates within a framework which ensures co-ordination of care across the population. Compassionate as well as efficient and effective provision of personal health services requires a solid foundation in primary care, with co-ordination, continuity, comprehensiveness, access and accountability. Links to public health[2] and community based organizations are essential. The stability of this link offers the best chance of realizing the vision of promoting both the individual's and the population's health.

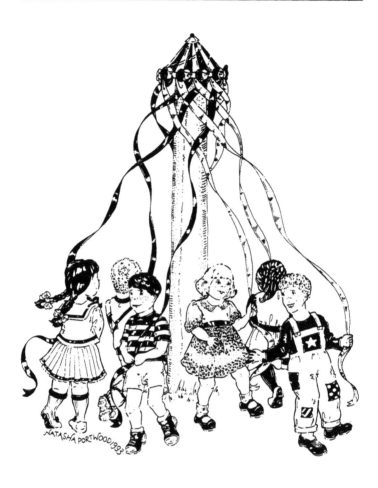

**Figure 3** The NHS merry-go-round.

The current emphasis on primary care led purchasing, be it through fundholding or locality commissioning largely ignores the provider functions of the professionals working in primary care teams. In future, it seems probable that there will be more provision of care in the community, more responsibilities, and consequently more resources for which to account. We need to debate the most appropriate mechanism for managing and co-ordinating such extended provision[3], recognizing that in addition the provider professionals will continue to commission consequential care.

Care for the home-based population has historically been provided by two distinct arms of the health service, the community services and primary care contractor services. The cultural differences between these two services belie their interdependence.

Community services, with their roots in local authority and local health authority services encompassing district nursing, health visiting, chiropody, physiotherapy, child health services, family planning, dietetics and frequently psychiatric services, are funded through Hospital and Community Health Services (HCHS) funds and are now mostly managed as separate NHS Community Trusts. Traditionally they have been organized on a geographically defined population basis, but they work closely with primary care teams and their registered lists.

Primary care contractor services such as GPs, opticians and dentists are self-employed and are in contract with the NHS. Their funding has historically been through a separate allocation for general medical services and while their contracts have been administered centrally (by the FHSA) their management has been mostly autonomous. Their development and organization has been focused on the individual registered patient.

## Background

This historic separation of services, structures, finance, management and perspective has led to inefficiency, duplication of services and is not in the patients' interest[4]. There is no market and no competition between the sectors because there is no incentive to change; rather, competition within primary care and between it and community units tends to fragment provision rather than co-ordinate it.

Community units co-ordinate and manage network organizations which enable the provision of flexible skilled services to the community without the necessity of extensive capital investment. Separation of the units from acute hospitals has protected their budget from predation by emergency services and thus enabled the development and expansion of important but less glamorous services, such as community drug teams, services for those with learning difficulties and community services for the elderly. The provision of community services requires specialist as well as expert generalist skills and all need support, development and education to maintain quality in a network environment. Increasingly, co-ordination of such support and education is occurring between Community Trusts and primary care, for example practice and community nurse training.

In the last 30 years, investment in primary care, both through training and premises development has been considerable. The majority of practices are now equipped to accept responsibilities and resources beyond traditional GMS funding, while NHS Community Trusts have seen their responsibilities reducing as services are either accepted as part of normal GP services (family planning and child surveillance) or are developed as outreach services from Acute Trusts (specialist nursing).

The pressure on GPs to provide a wider range of services needs to be monitored. Their role as the expert generalist is vital to the health service but is threatened by:

- increasing patient demand, some of which is inappropriate

- increasing service responsibilities for commissioning and providing a wider range of services, such as child surveillance and minor surgery

- pressure on finances which compels further service development simply to maintain profitability, many practices feel they are having to run faster to stand still

- the demand for greater accountability which confronts the constraints of a national contract and all the historic independent culture enshrined in the Red Book and GMSC.

This chapter suggests extending the contracting framework of the NHS so as to co-ordinate primary and community provider services and introduce incentives through competition and quality assurance. In line with recent health service policy[5] purchasing of care is primary care led. In 1996 Health Authorities (analogous to American Regional Health Alliances) will have strategic development roles, monitor and support providers and facilitate service development. The Primary Care Trust (comparable with the American Ambulatory Care Centre) should provide the framework necessary to tackle issues, such as in the inverse care law, which have proved so resistant to treatment in the past[6].

Implicit in the description of this model is the assumption that primary care led purchasing will precipitate the development of a culture of co-operation and co-ordination (Figure 1 style) as a response to the fragmentary tendency in extended fundholding. We already see supra-practice co-operation through developments such as multi-funds and night co-operatives and this tendency will receive a boost as the balance of forces moves away from maintaining small partnerships towards organizational development. The requirement for greater accountability; the necessity for policy to be drawn from a broader consensus; the necessity for buffering financial risk against population size; the desire of all sides for a redefinition of the contract between doctor and patient and the requirement for extended skills in the community, inherent in devolution of care from the hospital, all point in this direction. As we move towards primary care led purchasing over the next few years the focus of Health Authorities will change towards monitoring, commissioning and developing primary and community care. They will push for co-ordination so as to promote cohesion in the provision of care and will challenge primary care partnerships to demonstrate credible governance, the transfer of HCHS resources will depend on the response.

# The proposed Primary Care Trust

The proposed unit can be formed by the merger of the provider functions of independent contractor partnerships and the community unit. It is anticipated that the new unit or Trust would also control most resources for purchasing secondary care services and be accountable to a Health Authority for performance. The relationship between the Community Trust and existing primary care provider units will need to evolve because the units are very diverse and need help to develop as effective organizations if they are to strengthen the Trust. Ideally, practitioners will become members of the Trust and receive a share of the profits but for others a salaried option would be appropriate and some partnerships might look for an affiliated membership as an alternative interim step.

This then is a Trust in the independent sector, the independent contractor status is maintained and strengthened through access to combined GMS and HCHS resources but controlled through a co-ordinated framework of local contracting. The model is more akin to a golf club than a hospital Trust. The management is largely in the hands of the members, there are various categories of membership, rights and responsibilities are inherent in membership and a central clubhouse function to support the network of core activities by the membership is developed; there might even be a club professional giving lessons and running a shop. The Trust's relationship with the Health Authority is analogous to a college within a university where responsibility for admissions, regulation, education and management rest with the college but the university co-ordinates strategy and monitors the market. Colleges compete for students and resources, so will Trusts. Co-operation between practices as part of fundholding Consortia and night co-operatives has shown that GPs can work together and it may well be that a number of partnerships will merge their purchaser and provider functions with the community unit as a preliminary step to full organizational integration. An alternative to meet the population's needs could mean the

Trust directly employing salaried GPs, (as is current practice in special circumstances), which might be an attractive option to doctors wishing to restrict their responsibilities and to Trusts wishing to address particular population needs, especially when they are unpredictable or unusually variable. Holiday areas, inner city and university areas are examples.

## The services to be provided by a Primary Care Trust

On the basis of a contract with the Health Authority or Commission for the full range of services to be provided direct or purchased through contracts with other providers the Primary Care Trust's range might include those services listed in Table 11.1. A possible management structure is shown in Table 11.2. The management team and the organization framework into which they fit are shown in Figure 4.

There will also be a need for external audit and evaluation of value for money and quality as part of an accountability framework, either through the Audit Commission, as with fundholding, or by another appropriate external agency.

**Table 11.1**   The possible range of services provided by the Primary Care Trust

---

*Provider services*

- General medical services, in competition with private sector independent practices

- Child health services

- Family planning services

- Health visiting

- Primary and community nursing

---

**Table 11.1** *continued*

- Community paramedical support professions

    Dietetics

    Physiotherapy

    Chiropody

    OT

- Dental services ⎫
- Opticians services ⎬ In competition with the private independent sector
- Pharmacy services ⎭

*Additional services agreed with the HA*

- Disability aids ⎫
- Psychiatric services ⎬ In competition with secondary care trust
- Learning difficulty services ⎪
- Maternity services ⎭

- Specialist service either directly provided or bought in (eg specialist nursing, community drug teams and community mental health teams)

*Purchasing function*

- GP services from primary care teams within the Trust (where practices opt to remain independent they would contract with the Health Authority direct)

- Secondary care services on behalf of the population, using the information, knowledge and experience of GPs and public health

**Table 11.1** *continued*

*Management services*

- Employment
- Training
- Audit
- Quality assurance
- Contracting
- Finance
- Administration
- Information on performance

**Table 11.2** Possible management structure

*Members*

- Shareholders
- Professional members (eg medical, dental)
- Corporate members' affiliated practices
- Honorary members

*Trust Board*

- Chair
- Chief executive
- Finance
- Public health
- Professional provider
- Medical director

**Table 11.2** *continued*

- Deputy medical director
- Members by election for Primary Care Team (PCTs)
- Non-executive or patient representative

*Health Policy Board*

- Chief executive
- Finance
- Public health
- GPs from PCTs concerned
- Nursing representatives
- Paramedic services
- CHC representative
- Social Services representative

*Ownership Board*

- Local Authority
- University
- Voluntary groups
- Professional groups
- Health Authority non-executive
- Acute Trust
- Trust Chief Executive and other directors

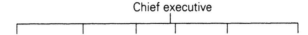

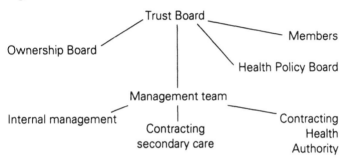

Organizational framework:

**Figure 4** Possible management team.

Within this context the key problems to be faced are discussed below.

### Ownership of capital

GP premises, capital and pensions could represent a barrier to organizational development. Perhaps allowing equity to be transferred into the capital value of the new Trust might be appropriate.

### Flexibility

The Trust will need to operate within the contracting framework of the NHS and will undoubtedly lose some of the flexibility of GP partnerships. It is envisaged that individual primary care teams would retain flexibility of response within agreed limits to match their interests and the agreed needs of the population they serve.

### Management skills

There are different types of management skills within community units and primary care. Mergers will require retraining of both to provide a third set of skills, this particularly applies to nursing services at present but will be even more relevant as the managing of GPs is addressed.

### Co-ordination
As with any locality based organization, boundary issues will cause difficulties with co-ordination as will boundaries between professions, such as that between practice nursing and district nursing.

### Democratic deficit
There will need to be a local ownership forum for the Trust, to provide it with a broader based perspective to inform policy development and as a mechanism for developing accountability to the community.

### Relationship with social services
There may need to be a combined policy board so that the increasing number of issues with links to both health and social services can be considered together.

### Links to GP-led purchasing and fundholding
Merger into a Primary Care Trust might evolve from fundholding, but does envisage the end of the personal incentives to make savings and could be seen as a curtailment of fundholding freedoms and independence.

### Competition
The Trust would compete with independent providers and, if boundaries overlap, with other Trusts. In addition they would compete for services with the acute sector. Will this be sufficient to improve provider performance?

### Freedom of choice versus planning
To what extent should the individual's right to choose his own GP and the GP's right to choose his patient be constrained within the Trust's right to plan services?

### Locality size

There will need to be defined boundaries either by practice or locality. In order to balance risk, given the resources involved, it might be that populations of about 50 000 would be appropriate, meaning there might be 6–10 per Commission and about 30 GPs in 10 practices. Inevitably there will be boundary and market issues to consider but these are not unique to this model. There is a need for an economic evaluation of the relationship between risk and population size, remembering that random variation can be a problem in small populations and loss of patient and contracting sensitivity a problem in large populations. The Trust will be too small to provide all services in house. Specialist incontinence and drugs advisory services, for example, will need to be brought in under contract.

Before considering the strengths and weaknesses of the Primary Care Trust model the context within which it has evolved needs consideration.

# Changing times

Any developing provider organization in the community has to reflect the needs of the community it is to serve. External or social factors influencing development include:

- demography
- technology
- patient empowerment
- mobility.

The population is ageing and the proportion of taxpayers declining. The family structure is changing with an increase in the number of single parent families and a decrease in the population of families with local grandparents and extended family support. What is the place of the family doctor in the post-family society?

Changes in health technology mean that patients need to spend less time in hospital and more episodes of care can be provided in the home setting. Shorter length of stay in hospital after surgery as a result of new anaesthetic and surgical techniques and the developments of less invasive investigation and treatment, such as endoscopy, increase the proportion of health care which can be undertaken within the community setting.

A central plank of recent policy has been to empower the individual. This means that individuals should have access to information to make their own informed decisions. A consequence of patient education and the development of patient charters has been a questioning of the traditional doctor/patient relationship. A rising number of complaints against professionals has been a reflection of this.

Continuity of care where the patient's family doctor would look after him from birth until retirement is no longer the norm. A mobile population means a different community network and the individuals within it require a different pattern of support.

Similarly the internal or organizational factors influencing development include the following.

- Devolution of care: Increasingly hospital services are focusing on the acutely sick. High technology care and specialist services mean less dependence on hospital beds.

- Care of elderly: The chronically sick are being transferred into the community where responsibility for their care is increasingly a drain on their personal savings, GMS, the community unit's resources and social services.

- DHA/FHSA mergers: The 1996 merger of Health Authorities will inevitably lead to consideration of the merger of different funding streams and budgets. Looking at resources in a more holistic fashion should encourage efficiency.

- Purchasing: The purchaser/provider separation and the introduction of local contracts for large parts of the NHS has implications for the future of those excluded from the local framework.

- Public health: There has been a rise in the importance of public health issues as opposed to personal health issues. Such issues as health promotion and disease prevention, the concentration on health of the nation priorities (eg HIV and AIDS, screening and cancer prevention, evidence based practice and efficiency) all require skills from public health to be widely available within the community[6]. Unfortunately, public health expertise has not yet been concentrated on primary care. This needs to change.

As a consequence the response so far to these social and organizational forces has been to promote the GP as the patient's agent and delegate control of resources as close to the patient as possible. This plays to the strengths of primary care but has led to fragmentation of provision and commissioning and ignores the weaknesses of the current structure. The strengths of current primary care organization are:

- flexibility: the ability to respond appropriately to change in circumstance

- independence: freedom of action to retain credibility with patients

- security: the ability to make long-term plans

- registered list: knowing where responsibility lies

- continuity of care: seeing care as part of life-style

- access: the availability of local expertize

- national contract: a framework for ensuring equity of access to resources across the country.

The weaknesses of the current structure are listed in Figure 5.

- The lack of accountability from primary care on performance and use of resources.

- Isolation: Primary Care Teams are not only independent but are also isolated from the rest of the health service both managerially and culturally.

- Separate budgets: Lack of a definition of GMS has meant that work can be devolved into primary care and GMS budget without resources. This haemorrhage hits practice profitability and damages morale.

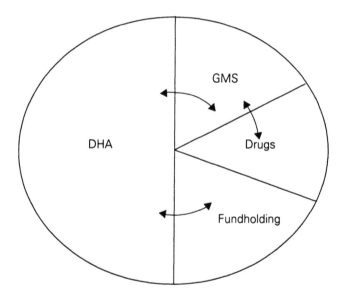

- Partnership problems: Unfortunately in any small long-term partnership the differences between partners both in terms of values and power can produce behaviour which is detrimental to patient care.

**Figure 5**  Weakness of the current structure.

- Cultural differences: Practice performance will reflect the values of the partnership and the national contract is too weak to control poor performance effectively.

- Inverse care law: The national contract has been unable to restrict the drift of resources away from areas of greatest need.

- Inverse profitability law: The national contract has also been unable to recompense extra effort adequately . It remains the case that the most profitable practices are frequently those which invest the least.

- Democratic deficit: The narrow policy-making board in primary care reflects only medical expertise and ignores the perspective of the other professionals concerned about the health needs of the population. The population's view is also under-represented, not a problem if GPs are adequately interpreting the needs of the population but very much an issue if their own priorities are different[7].

- Governance weakness: The isolation and independence of primary care exposes teams to the accusation that they lack openness, integrity and accountability and that there is too great a potential for misappropriation of public funds for the public to have complete confidence that it is safe to channel the majority of NHS resources through them.

- Management weakness: Primary care management has evolved with primary care teams and like them frequently lacks breadth of vision, skills and capacity. The separation of GP continuing education from staff training and the rest of NHS training inhibits change in this area[8].

**Figure 5**  *continued.*

If current policies concentrate on the strengths and ignore the weaknesses of the current position then the Primary Care Trust needs to address those weaknesses. However, through co-ordination a new dynamic can be developed offering the following opportunities:

- control over resources
- patient centred decision-making
- career structure
- skill substitution
- professional quality assurance

There is no doubt that co-operation between practices serving a local community and the community unit serving that population would mean that there would be a powerful alliance for the provision of expanded services.

An expanded policy-making board should challenge medical dominance and facilitate a broader community approach to health issues, allowing patient-centred decision-making to become more common.

The public health perspective is important for such a community health service and can be more adequately represented as an important contributor to the changed perspective.

There are great opportunities for improving the efficiency of health care provision through re-engineering the service as a consequence of merging, for example, nursing policies and child health surveillance policies[9].

There is a great need for professional development programmes, training and career support within primary care. At present, staff and practitioners are isolated from full pension and training rights. Inter-practice co-operation could facilitate access to this. In addition, career development opportunities for GPs would be promoted.

Efficiency and cost-effectiveness arguments would encourage an expansion of the trend to skill substitution through further delegation to nurse-practitioners, triage nursing in primary care and expansion of nursing auxiliary provision in the community. This could liberate doctors to practise medicine. Fundholding has already illustrated some potential for re-engineering patient services but this model will really drive efficiency in the community through re-engineering and skill substitution by replacing incentives for improved efficiency for perverse incentives leading to rationing of resources and care.

The Trust will need to monitor the quality of its services and the Health Authority will only contract with it if quality is assured. The Trust will need to develop a matrix of quality assessments including elements similar to American medical staff bylaws but also incorporating the British experience of quality in primary care[10]. The alternative of a separate 'Utilization Review Organization' as a provider accreditation mechanism would be a costly irrelevance.

There are, however, threats to cohesion in the model. There is no doubt that transfer of responsibility without resources is damaging the profitability of many primary care teams and stretching the resources of many community units. Without the community services having control over the resource allocation policy then such dumping endangers the quality, motivation and success of community health service. Enhanced provider co-operation without purchasing responsibilities in the community and without merger of GMS and HCHS funding does nothing to prevent dumping of care between providers. Unless the Trust is within the local contracting framework and able both to provide services and purchase care it will just be a bigger dumping ground than current primary care.

Current trends towards providing care under protocols and guidelines helps to make practices more accountable for performance and helps to develop a quality assurance mechanism. However, this trend may also limit the individual's freedom to diverge from normal accepted behaviour.

Management costs in primary care have historically been small. An increase in management does not necessarily mean more effective management and there will be a great need for investment in training both to manage and to be managers[11]. Current concerns over the transaction costs involved in primary care led purchasing beg for an analysis of the policy and can provide the impetus for a cohesive model such as the proposed Primary Care Trust.

Current developments such as night co-operatives, emergency centres and fundholding Consortia all tend to reduce the proportion of contacts with the registered doctor. Within the Trust there will need to be safeguards to protect the doctor/patient relationship and ensure professional freedoms.

## The future

Bearing in mind the complex and inter-related issues discussed above there is a pressing need to develop this community care provider service within a framework that learns from the strengths and weaknesses of the current service and reflects the opportunities available and the perceived threats. Such a service needs to:

- learn from the community orientated primary care work from the King's Fund[12] where public health and GP perspectives can help to link service development to commissioning strategies

- be accountable to patients, to the community and to health service management for performance and use of resources

- respect the principles of corporate governance (eg openness, integrity and accountability)

- reflect the complexity of managing the professions involved in primary care by including them in the membership so that they 'own' the unit and work in partnership with management

- have the power within it and the control of resources necessary to re-engineer patient services internally and use its information and knowledge to be an effective purchaser of hospital services

- be of sufficient size to balance the risk of random variation in demand against the loss of freedom and direct control within small organizations

- have the freedom to transfer funding between budgets and to use resources either to provide the service themselves or to subcontract and purchase services from outside

- develop skills in financial management, contract management, training and the provision of such extended primary care services as nursing, counselling, physiotherapy, chiropody, dietetics and occupational therapy

- recognize that competition is a spur to effectiveness, either through developing overlapping 'localities' or by competition for purchasing authority (ie being an accredited purchaser as well as provider)

The strengths of the model are:

- improved co-ordination of care and policy development on provision of integrated service, nursing, family planning, child health services

- better use of skills (ie management, finance, public health)

- enhanced potential for skill substitution to improve efficiency

- quality assurance in primary care

- broader ownership of policy base

- primary care led purchasing with reduced risk

- mechanism for integrating GMS with HCHS

- support for isolated practitioners

- preservation of patient choice of family doctor

- maintenance of registered list, continuity of care, generalist filter and common record

- pool of FHSA experience available within new Health Authorities' development

- levers for tackling the inverse care law, locality sensitive contracting, public health perspective in primary care, and change to the incentives primary care teams have from focusing on demand to focusing on need.

The weaknesses of the model are:

- GP's loss of independence; issues of capital, employment status and partnership structure will need to be reviewed

- position of public health working with both purchaser and provider

- links between Trust and neighbours, boundary issues

- co-ordination of care between individual GP and consultant

- balance of size (resources) and issues of access

- competition in the market, currently it might be said that there is plenty of competition between practices and the community unit. In reality, competition is very restricted and has not been an efficient arbiter of change.

The model brings with it opportunities to:

- enhance the input of public health knowledge into community care

- manage the devolution of care rather than react to the antagonism it generates

- invest capital in primary care in a planned way, from the NHS or the private sector

- expand the career prospects for all the staff and bring primary care teams within the NHS employment framework.

In contrast it also brings threats to:

- the autonomy of the primary care teams
- the flexibility of the primary care teams
- primary/secondary care co-operation
- the power of professional interest groups to preserve inappropriate structures
- some Local Medical Committees
- incentives for GPs to invest in high quality premises and care
- subsidized growth in GP's pensions, via cost rent schemes.

## Conclusion

Current developments in the NHS are putting increasing pressures on the independent contractor status, GP partnerships and under-capitalized community units. Organizational development with merger between them to enhance skills, balance risk and provide access to resources will be essential. In addition, such merger and organizational development in Primary Care Trusts can enhance the acknowledgement of governance issues in the community and improve efficiency in the delivery of health care through the co-ordination of medical and nursing policies.

In future, patient care will be largely provided outside hospitals. Co-ordination of that care, leadership and the management of resources require the development of a new partnership between community care providers so that care teams can share patient centred objectives rather than focus on perverse incentives, cross budget dumping and historical mistrust of motives.

The health service is about the health of every individual in the population. We need to rise above factionalism and realize that change to community care provider arrangements is long overdue and essential if the role of the GP is to develop and play its part in providing appropriate health care as we set sail into the twenty-first century.

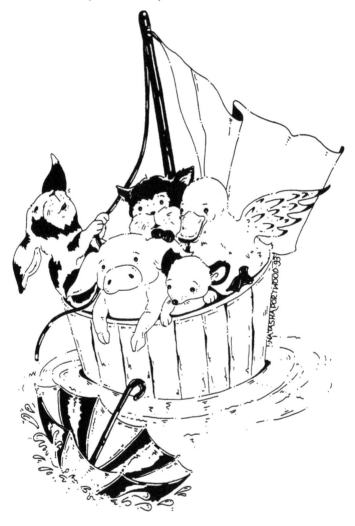

**Figure 6** Setting sail.

# References

1 Starfield B (1994) Is primary care essential? *The Lancet.* **344**: 1129–33.

2 Lee P R (1994) Models of excellence. *The Lancet.* **344**: 1484–6.

3 Light D W (1994) Managed care. *The Lancet.* **344**: 1197–9.

4 Murray S A (1995) How many general practitioners for 1433 patients? *BMJ.* **310**: 100.

5 National Health Service Executive (1994) EL (94) 79. *Developing NHS purchasing and GP fundholding.* NHSE, London.

6 Tudor-Hart J (1988) A new kind of doctor. Merlin, London.

7 Starey N, Bosanquet N and Griffiths J (1993) General practitioners in partnership with management: An organisational model for debate. *BMJ.* **306**: 308–10.

8 Pearson P and Jones K (1994) The primary health care non-Team? *BMJ.* **309**: 1387.

9 NHS Management Executive (1991) *Integrating primary and secondary health care.* HMSO, London.

10 Irvine D (1990) Managing for quality in general practice; Medical audit series. King's Fund Centre, London.

11 Huntington J (1995) Practice management: whose business? Radcliffe Medical Press, Oxford.

12 Williams S (1994) Community oriented primary care: from concept to reality. *Primary Care Management.* **4**: 3–6.

# Joint ventures: public and private collaboration in primary health care | 12

*Stuart Chidgey*

## NHS values

It is useful, from time to time, to remind ourselves of the defining and enduring values of the NHS. These values are that health care in this country is available, appropriate, accessible and acceptable and that it is free to the consumer at the point of delivery. This being the case, where in the NHS of the mid-1990s do we find the role of 'protector of the NHS'? Most would argue that this is the responsibility of politicians. Despite all the rhetoric there does remain a broad political consensus in support of these NHS values. Where there will always be political divergence is in the means by which they can best be safeguarded.

The NHSE, both centrally and through its regional offices, is given the task of ensuring that the NHS sustains these values and that health is delivered in the most cost-effective manner. Locally, the new Health Commissions (about to emerge in 1995/6 from the amalgamation of DHAs and FHSAs have their future role defined as: health strategy development; monitoring services to ensure that both national policy and local strategy are implemented effectively; and support for GPs in their role as purchasers through general practice fundholding, and providers of health and health care[1]. These roles are core

NHS responsibilities and as such should always remain in the public sector.

## Purchasing and providing health

The NHS reforms heralded in *Working for patients*[2], have led to a clarification of the roles and responsibilities of the purchasers of health (Health Commissions and GPFHs) and those of providers of secondary and community health care (NHS Trusts). The progress of the NHS reforms can be categorized within distinct stages. First, the separation of the purchaser and provider functions within DHAs and the establishment of NHS Trusts and GPFH. Second, attention was focused on the configuration of purchasing with both the amalgamation of a number of existing DHAs and their subsequent merger with FHSAs. Third, the restructuring of the provision of primary, community and secondary health care, which is currently underway. A constant theme of the reforms has been the development of GPFH as the preferred model for purchasing health. Attention is now turning, in the era of a primary care led NHS, to the question of the future configuration of the provision of primary care. Past distinctions are becoming untenable. There is a blurring of perceived boundaries between secondary, community and primary care. Such classifications will become increasingly meaningless as what we are interested in is the best quality health care, not where it happens to be delivered.

GPFHs find themselves in a unique position in the NHS, they have a responsibility to deliver both a purchaser and provider role; purchasing hospital and Community Health Services and providing primary care services. This split personality of general practices is reflected in the way these roles are treated by Health Commissions which have a dual relationship with GPFHs, they are resourced and monitored separately as purchasers and providers of health.

If the responsibility for purchasing what we generally understand to be primary care, (that is those services provided by GPs and PHCTs, is to be vested with Health Commissions, from 1996, how should we structure and resource the provision of primary care. It is becoming clear that there is unlikely to be one answer to this question, and that a variety of models will appear appropriate to local circumstances.

## Providing primary health care

Health Commissions, charged with the overall responsibility of assessing the health care needs of the local population and for ensuring that those needs are met, will inevitably begin to challenge existing configurations in the provision of primary care. For Commissions the key measures will be meeting targets in terms of for example, *Health of the nation* and *Patient charter* standards. The question for the Commission then becomes: how can we best manage the provision of primary care in our area to meet our objectives? Such a question is certain to leave the present structure of general practice and primary health care wanting in some areas. Already we are seeing a mixed economy in the provision of primary care. Who is best placed to deliver what the Commission requires, is it general practice, a Community NHS Trust, a charitable trust, a private sector provider or a combination of these?

At this stage it is important to distinguish between the GP in his professional role as a clinician providing general medical services and the GP partnership/practice as an entity being the organization responsible for providing primary health care to a defined population. The first will certainly continue, the second is less certain.

What could the new structure be and is there a role for the private sector? GPs have, in a sense, always been private providers of health. GPs are self-employed with a contract for services with the NHS, regulated currently in 1995 by FHSAs.

However, this has always been somewhat anomalous as the majority of GPs spend at least 90% of their time both working for and deriving their income from the NHS.

## Primary health care markets

Within Commissions the role of market maker is perceived as relatively new and little understood. The NHS does, however, have some experience of market making within the Family Health Services (eg GPs, community pharmacists, dentists and opticians). Currently the ability to enter a local market to provide these services is regulated by the NHS for GPs and community pharmacists but not for dentists or opticians. As far as GPs are concerned, the Medical Practices Committee controls GP provision by its classification of areas as: designated (ie under-doctored), open, intermediate or restricted (over-doctored). Similarly the establishment of a community pharmacy must be proved to be both necessary and desirable for an NHS application to dispense to be granted. As far as dentists and opticians are concerned, the market is far less fettered; suitably qualified practitioners can set up shop and will either flourish or founder based on their ability to attract custom.

At present, GPs and NHS Trusts are both protected as the monopoly suppliers of NHS General Medical and Community Nursing Services. Should a purchaser be dissatisfied with either service his options for going elsewhere are highly circumscribed and limited to other NHS providers.

For GMS the market has been highly controlled and regulated. While few would argue for a complete deregulation of access to the GMS market this does not mean that the GP partnership should maintain a monopoly as the only legitimate organizational model for the provision of primary care.

# GP partnerships

The GP partnership is already feeling the strains of the reorientation of the focus of the NHS from a secondary to a primary care led service. GPs are the first to admit to overload as they endeavour to meet ever increasing patient expectation for primary care services at the same time as NHS policy gives them increased control and responsibility for NHS resources. This relatively new commissioning role has been loaded onto a structure that also has an exiting responsibility for the running of the practice, a medium sized business unit.

Innovative practices are already circumventing the rules, and while the GP partnership remains the official legal entity, scratch the surface of some practices and you will find quite different organizations. Co-existing with the partnership are examples of Consortia arrangements with other practices, collaboration with the NHS Community Trusts, limited liability companies, separate property owning partnerships, and public/private alliances. These organizational forms are responses to the sometimes conflicting demands of what a modern general practice is. How long can a range of increasingly diverse roles co-exist within one organizational form without splitting at the seams? For how long should we ask a GP practice to be a provider of primary health care, a purchaser of acute and secondary health and an independent business? A practice has to fulfil the rules of purchaser (core public), provider (mixed market public/private) and business (private).

Many organizations, both in the public and private sectors, are focusing on their core business activity and divesting themselves of non-core activity. The core business of general practice has traditionally been the provision of primary care. Loading immense purchaser responsibilities onto an organization structured for its historical activity will inevitably lead to, what we are beginning to witness in many cases, the breakdown of the traditional general practice as the organizational model and its replacement by a number of hybrids.

## Private provision of primary care

Could what we are seeing be the emergence of what is in a sense a market within a market? While GPs will continue to contract direct with Health Commissions, the actual provision of many primary care services will be in the hands of both public and private sector organizations. Indeed, the whole concept of there being a distinction between public and private providers is becoming irrelevant. What matters is that the service is delivered to the patients free at the point of delivery and that it is available, appropriate, accessible and acceptable.

While the private sector is prevented from contracting directly with a Commission for the provision of GMS (unlike hospital services), it can enter partnership arrangements with general practices, Health Commissions and NHS Trusts. The co-operation on combined capital investment between GP and retail pharmacists is becoming increasingly a characteristic of modern multi-purpose health centres in such locations as Minehead in Somerset and Ferndown in Dorset.

The first and obvious example of partnership arrangements is in the field of primary care facilities, such as buildings and equipment. Standards in the provision of premises for primary care differ greatly throughout the country. Among the poorest provision is where GPs and PHCTs are housed in Health Centres in the ownership of either Commissions or Trusts. In addition, inner city practice accommodation is generally accepted to be of poor quality.

The traditional source of funding for the development of primary care premises has been through GMS Cost Rent and Improvement Grant Schemes. However, access to these funds has been restricted over recent years at the same time as there has been an inability of these schemes to fund the development of the facilities required in the era of a primary care led NHS.

Private developers are already entering partner arrangements with innovative general practices to share the investment costs of new facilities. A further step is where private sector partnerships are developed to introduce private sector capital, skills and experience into the design, building and management of premises. This should not cross the GP independent contractor relationship with the Health Commission. The property owners would receive rent from the GPs, and could utilize space in the premises for related health services. A possible development of this is for a general practice to contract out its management and administration support roles. The GPs continuing to provide GMS while support functions could effectively be in the hands of a professional management agency. Precedents for this have already been established where there exists a contractual arrangement between a practice and a private sector management agency to manage fundholding on behalf of the practice.

A second and rapidly developing area of public and private sector collaboration in primary care is where GPs, especially GPFHs, contract with private health providers to provide a range of services in a primary care setting. As we shift the balance of health from secondary to primary settings, discreet areas of service provision, often hitherto provided in hospitals can be provided in primary care. NHS Trusts have been slow off the mark in offering such services in primary care; not so the private sector. An example is the provision of day case surgery as provided by EMP Ltd at the Old Cottage Hospital Surgery in Epsom, Surrey. Other services where a number of private providers are actively marketing their services to fundholders include pathology, radiology, physiotherapy, chiropody and osteopathy.

A third collaborative opportunity arises from concepts of Pharmacy Benefit Management and Disease Management, ideas that have their origin in the US health care system. Such schemes are being pioneered by such multi-national pharmaceutical companies as Glaxo and Merck Sharp & Dohme seeking to redefine their business away from that of being the supplier of pills to that of being partners with the NHS in the provision of health. Although such partner arrangements will need to be carefully scrutinized to ensure they meet the principles on which the NHS is based, and also offer value for money to the NHS, it is likely that there will be added value for the NHS.

Organizations such as BUPA, Healthcall, commercial banks and retail pharmacy multiples are interested in partnering GPs and Health Commissions in primary care developments. They are likely to be supplemented in the future by pharmaceutical companies and companies such as EMP Ltd which aim to develop a number of day case facilities within primary care settings. The Private Finance Initiative now supports such developments as private sector operators are encouraged to fund, design, manage and build health care facilities for the NHS. Minor Injuries Centres and Out of Hours services are two obvious examples of such facilities as the national GMS contract restrictions are loosened.

The trends described above can be illustrated by reference to an example of a primary care provider which was maximizing its potential for collaboration with the private sector. Although this is a hypothetical example, the author is aware of practices which are operating with one or more of the arrangements described.

This general practice has developed its premises under the auspices of a limited liability company. Some, but not all, of the partners have established the company with non-medical directors who can bring capital and business management skills to develop the premises. The company owns and manages the facilities and has a lease with the GP practice which is reimbursed expenses via the FHSA, in the same way as other practices. The surgery is state-of-the-art with facilities for the extended PHCT. The company has separate leases for a pharmacy, day case surgery provider, pathology and X-ray providers and consulting rooms for physiotherapy and chiropody. These services are provided by the private sector, but are free at the point of delivery to the consumer. They are purchased by fundholders and Health Commissions.

What this example seeks to illustrate is the range of possibilities for collaboration between the NHS and the private sector in primary care. They will not be appropriate in some circumstances. What needs to be recognized is that a fundamental restructuring of the way health is delivered is occurring. Traditional categorizations of secondary/community/ primary care and public/private are becoming irrelevant; they are the province of health professionals not the users of the service. What the NHS consumer of health requires is best quality health care, free at the point of delivery.

## Conclusion

This chapter has attempted to explore four key themes:

- in a publicly funded health system such as the NHS the purchasing of health is a core public sector function as it is performed on behalf of the public

- it is for the newly established Health Commissions to regulate the primary care provider market

- the providing of health is a mixed economy of public and private (and voluntary) sectors. Private providers are established in both the hospital and long-term care markets. However, the provision of primary health care is restricted to GPs, structured as partnerships and with other members of PHCTs

- we are likely to witness greater collaboration between NHS providers of primary care (GPs and PHCTs) and privately funded health organizations.

As we manage the shift in the balance of health from secondary to primary and community settings, more and more services that are currently delivered in hospitals will be delivered in primary care centres. Some of these services the GP will continue to provide, for others the GP will act in his role as purchaser and the private sector will provide them.

In either case it will be for health purchasers as Commissioners or GPFHs to articulate health needs, translate these needs into contracts and monitor performance. Quality is everybody's business and standards must be maintained.

We are likely to see a development of the mixed market for primary care provision. This chapter has attempted to explain the rationale and opportunities for partnerships with the private sector. Future providers of primary care could equally be Community Trusts, charitable trusts, and voluntary or commercial organizations.

## References

1   National Health Service Executive (1994) EL(94)79. *Developing NHS purchasing and GP fundholding.* NHSE, London.

2   Department of Health (1989) *Working for patients.* HMSO, London.

# Primary managed care: the Lyme alternative   | 13

*Barry Robinson*

Influenced heavily by the reported success of American Health
Maintenance Organizations (HMO) in delivering complete
managed care packages[1], the integration of health and social
care to provide a seamless service to the public has now become
a part of the UK 'dream' as well. As a result, in 1995, strategic
planning authorities, including Health Authorities, FHSAs,
SSDs and the Department of Health, are striving to develop
joint commissioning as the means of integrating and co-ordinating the planning of all care. Perhaps because of the differing agenda of these authorities and, of course, the diverse
sources of funding, such co-ordination can be difficult in the
absence of unified HMO style organizational arrangements.
There are many examples of good local practice where
strategic planning authorities are drawing more closely together and devising joint action plans in specific areas of care,
but there remain many areas where such integration is only a
remote inspiration.

There is, nevertheless, considerable political and managerial interest in the concept of joint commissioning as DHAs
and FHSAs draw closer together, and various models for integrating health and social care authorities have been proposed.
Some favour a return to the provision of health and social care
services by local authorities with their locally elected and
accountable members, while others see in Health Commis-

sions an opportunity to manage the health and social care agenda more effectively. Few seem to have considered a rather more radical approach which requires less major structural and organizational change, yet has the potential to deliver an enhanced and integrated service to the public.

This approach can be termed primary managed care, the model for which has been developed over the last three years in Lyme Regis, Dorset. This chapter, developed from Robinson[2], sets out its philosophy and organization and argues that this US-initiated development could, if properly customized, have the potential for widespread use by UK general practice.

## The local context

Lyme Regis lies at the far south-western tip of Dorset, with a community that extends across the boundary into east Devon. The locality, consisting of approximately 8000 patients, is served by two general practices; a single-handed practitioner, and a group practice of four. One-third of all the patients are resident within Devon with a different FHSA, DHA and SSD. The secondary care providers in health care are all situated some 25 miles distant from Lyme Regis at Taunton, Yeovil, Exeter and Dorchester, while the area offices for social services are located some 10 miles away at Bridport (Dorset) and Honiton (Devon). The headquarters of the SSDs are situated within the county towns at Exeter and Dorchester, much further away.

The Lyme Community Care Unit was founded in April 1992 to provide a common-sense solution to the provision of an integrated health and social care service to all citizens living within the locality, regardless of their address or GP. Among the tasks which the Unit set itself, in its original business plan, was to translate this confusing and complex web of service providers and purchasers into a single organizational model whose care was centred on the citizen, while it retained accountability to the statutory agencies.

With the status of a limited company, the Unit was set up by the GPs working within the locality, but it is an independent and separate entity whose remit is declared within its mission statement:

> 'The business of the Lyme Community Care Unit is to improve health and well being by the provision of high quality, comprehensive, integrated patient-orientated health and social services to all those living within the locality. Wherever practical, these services should combine to optimize the quality of life for residents by providing appropriate care in, or as close as possible to, their own home'.

# The Unit's philosophy

Before discussing the organizational process which underpins the operation of the Lyme Community Care Unit, it is important to consider the fundamental philosophy on which the Unit is based.

We believe that we are faced with a remorseless rise in the demand for care in the face of static or diminishing resources. The demographic changes and the rapid economic development of third world countries are forcing change upon us. Governments grapple with the complex task of containing health and social care costs through various organizational models. Healthcare Reform Bills in the USA, the advent of fundholding and the provider–purchaser split in the UK, and the Oregon experiment in prioritizing health care[3] are but a few of the many initiatives which serve this common aim. These are all important and yet perhaps fail to address the central issue.

The primary managed care paradigm requires that only the citizen, as part of the wider community, can effectively constrain his or her own demand for increasing levels of care. Responsibility for health and social well being must primarily be a personal one. It is the duty of governments and their agencies to facilitate the maintenance of health and then to ensure that adequate and appropriate provision is made when individual effort is not sufficient. It is this fundamental shift in responsibility, from government and its organizations to the citizens and their communities, which marks the Lyme Community Care Unit as a radical innovation.

The second premise which underlines the operation of the Unit is that, where appropriate, citizens would always prefer care to be provided in or as close as possible to their own homes. This maxim underlies our contracting process and ensures that, for each service, we constantly question whether it could be provided more effectively and more appropriately within the locality. It may be summed up as a paraphrase of our mission statement 'Do locally what you properly can and then buy from others what you cannot do'.

The third platform for our enterprise is the principle that the total financial resource available to a community should be transparent. Top-slicing, special projects and other such initiatives lead, we believe, to the citizen failing to understand that there is a finite resource available for health and social care. If the totality is made transparent and available, then decisions about utilization, including the setting of priorities, can be made by the community. Consensus within the community will decide operational policy, informed by expert advice and national and regional strategic directions.

The fourth and final support for our business is the principle that most of us wish to enjoy our daily work. A simple observation, but one that has been sadly neglected within the NHS and SSDs in the past. Specialist training and the willingness to let expensively acquired skills wither through disuse had led, in our view, to a workforce which fails to utilize fully its many skills, to the detriment of both citizen and carers alike.

# Building a generic team

From the beginning, we believed that the establishment of a generic workforce, utilizing all those skills which had been gained at such expense and personal difficulty, should be employed to work within the Lyme Community Care Unit. Workers' boundaries would be defined by their professional accountability to themselves and the public, and they would be expected to draw on expert professional advice and assistance whenever appropriate. All staff would be directly employed by the Unit, wherever possible, not seconded, nor merely liaising with the team.

The analogy with the GP is obvious, and it should be remembered that general practice, for all its failings, has provided one of the successes of the NHS since its inception in 1946. The twin pillars of gate-keeping to specialist services and generic working mean that most of us in the UK feel confident in the relationship which we have developed with our GP. We trust his or her ability to deal on a day-to-day basis with our health-care problems, confident that the GP has access to the specialist care required if local skills or facilities are inadequate.

The Lyme Community Care Unit accordingly developed a business plan which postulated that it was necessary to develop a strong, comprehensive and motivated primary care agency which incorporated both health and social care professionals working together with the citizens. The Unit is the employer of a wide range of community staff, and operates a hospital-at-home scheme. If care is to be transferred to the community, we deem it essential that there is in place a structure for delivering standards of care comparable with those which can be found in secondary care providers. The professionals and areas which are represented within the team employed by the Lyme Community Care Unit and working within the community are:

- community nursing

- hospital-at-home
- physiotherapy
- occupational therapy
- social worker
- chiropody
- casualty
- health visiting
- dietitian
- speech therapy
- community psychiatric nurse
- school nurse
- counsellor
- GPs
- care managers
- midwife
- community health advisor.

Job descriptions were written by the staff within three months of being offered a contract of employment with the Unit. Behind this was the intention to emphasize the personal responsibility of the professionals to utilize their skills, and the needs of their particular client group, to develop their service.

Perhaps for too long, job descriptions in statutory agencies have been the lowest common denominator, designed to ensure that mistakes do not occur and that litigation is not a problem. Instead, we need our colleagues to be free to exercise their skills in order that care can be improved and costs contained.

# Involving the community

To achieve our primary objective, transferring responsibility for health and social well being from the statutory bodies to the citizen, we have a management advisory group. This representative body is nominated by health and social care professionals working within the locality. Alongside these lay members sit elected health and social care professionals and a general practice representative from each of the practices. The Unit general manager completes this management advisory group as the single executive member and the conduit for decisions from the advisory group to the Unit management team. One of the GPs acts part-time as Unit general manager.

Although the practices involved in the Unit are not fundholders, one of the principles underlying general practice fundholding has been that the GP is able to act as a competent and informed patient advocate. We would broadly support this view, and experience teaches that such an informed advocate purchases sensibly and effectively on behalf of his or her patients. In an ideal world, we may wish to transfer responsibility back to each individual, perhaps by a voucher system for health and social care, but practicalities and service planning make such a development unlikely, at least in the foreseeable future.

While accepting the valued role of GPs as patients' advocates, we felt that we could introduce more personal responsibility for patients' health and social well being. The management advisory group acts as both the ears and voice of the community. As voice, it is intended to inform the Unit management team of the needs, wishes and hopes of the citizens within this community; as ears, we trust that it will take back and disseminate the message that resources are finite, that the responsibility for health and well being rests with the citizen and that, when these fail, the Unit has made provision in accordance with their wishes.

Thus far then, the Unit is working towards achieving its primary aims of transferring care to the citizen and providing appropriate generic care within the locality through the team of professional and non-professional staff employed directly. However, we are all aware that this local or community expenditure represents only a small fraction of the total expenditure on health and social care.

## Acting as purchasing agent

The major portion of expenditure still goes on residential or secondary health care providers, often at distant centres. The Lyme Community Care Unit now has available to it the total health care budget previously held by the Dorset Health Commission and East and North Devon Health Authority on behalf of our residents. The Unit acts as purchasing agent for these two authorities and all contracts are negotiated and monitored through our own team. The remit is to purchase appropriate and timely secondary care which complements local provision but does not seek to replace it. This is locality purchasing of health care, based on needs identified by Unit staff in conjunction with patients and the wider community.

Early in 1995, agreement was reached with both Devon and Dorset SSDs for the Unit to become the care managers for citizens resident within the area. After appropriate staff training, the Lyme Community Care Unit became the first cross-boundary agency in the country to manage the total health and social care expenditure for a defined population. The opportunities are obvious to all those who have responsibility for delivering care. We believe that significant benefits flow from such an integrated approach in terms of delivering comprehensive, integrated, value-for-money care.

The Lyme Community Care Unit acknowledges that each of its statutory commissioning authorities has a different agendum. In part, these are fashioned from central directives and policy initiatives, while funding arrangements and local accountability will also play their part. Neither do we forget the different backgrounds that health and social care professionals bring to their work. However, are these differing agenda of any significant interest to the citizen who needs information and education to maintain personal well being and then appropriate and planned professional care when self-care is not sufficient? Alternatively, do these differing agenda confuse, confound and lead to a dependency culture in which only the professionals are deemed to have sufficient knowledge or expertize to manage the affairs of the citizen? We respect the rights of authorities to their own strategic objectives which must inform our planning; but we serve our community, and that community has a right to expect local variation and accountability for the services which we provide.

## Conclusion

In summary, the Lyme Community Care Unit is a primary managed care agency committed to utilizing the available resources to the benefit of the community. It is founded on the principles that:

* responsibility for the maintenance of well being belongs to the citizen

* appropriate professional care should always be provided locally

* the total financial resource must be available and transparent

* caring staff should be fully valued and utilized.

Subject to an independent evaluation, the Unit welcomes the opportunity to demonstrate its successes and learn from informed debate.

At Lyme we enjoy our work, which has not been without difficulties. We believe in the primary managed care principles which underpin our daily activity. We look forward to the day when our community, composed of the individual citizens to whom we offer support, will fully exercise its duty for self-care. Illness and social need will always be with us, and we intend to offer the most appropriate care and support in these circumstances.

With the true individual ownership of the agenda and resources by our citizens, the managed primary care alternative offers general practice a way of building on its best traditions for personal care and business enterprise.

## References

1  Fry J and Horder J (1995) *Primary health care in an international context.* Nuffield, London, pp. 30–41.

2  Robinson B (1994) *Integrating Health and Social Care: The Lyme Community Care Unit in Community Care Management and Planning.* **2** (5): 139–43.

3  Honigsbaum F (1991) Who shall live? Who shall die? Oregon's health financing proposals. King's Fund College Papers No 4. King's Fund College, London.

# From invention to innovation

# 14

*June Huntington*

Peter Senge distinguishes between invention and innovation by describing:

> 'that cold, clear morning in December 1903, at Kitty Hawk, North Carolina when the fragile aircraft of Wilbur and Orville Wright proved that powered flight was possible. Thus was the airplane invented; but it would take more than thirty years before commercial aviation could serve the general public . . . Engineers say that a new idea has been "invented" when it is proven to work in the laboratory. The idea becomes an "innovation" only when it can be replicated reliably on a meaningful scale at practical cost'[1].

A range of primary care organizations is described in this book. They are the response some GPs and managers, but mainly GPs, have made to the challenge of producing a primary care led NHS. What made them possible and what will ensure that some or all will be sufficiently robust to be 'replicated on a meaningful scale at practical cost'?

# Clinical leadership

The introduction of a general management culture challenged the collusive, functionally specialized nature of NHS careers and reminded us that the capacity to bring about change was individual rather than occupational. Sir Roy Griffiths, who urged the application of general management principles to the NHS, observed that the closer the service came to the patient, the more appropriate it was for the doctor to manage it. From my own experience in leading management programmes for doctors, I conclude that most clinicians who move into managerial roles do so for several reasons:

- to achieve improvements to the service which elude them as individual clinicians

- to pursue the intellectual challenge of grasping and working with a system of greater size and complexity

- to address the ethical challenge of identifying a pattern of resource allocation that will offer the greatest value for each pound spent.

Many doctors enter general practice because they seek work that promises autonomy and independence. The contributors to this book describe working models of primary care provision and suggest that some GPs are now building unprecedented relationships with other professions and organizations. They have led, are leading, and want to continue to do so. They are shaping NHS 2000, now. Wisely, they see that this is the only way that they can secure the autonomy and independence commensurate with a publicly funded NHS. They have taken to heart the imperative: manage or you will be managed.

They have displayed individual creativity, vision, leadership and perseverance. What is less explicit, but well known to others who have been involved in the creation and development of these organization inventions, is that they are also the product of individuals-in-association. In an account of the development to the Lyme Community Care Unit[2], Barry Robinson testified to the support of Ian Carruthers, Chief Executive of Dorset Health Commission, in the development of the organization.

I have at times heard the Lyme unit, described in Chapter 13, referred to as 'Barry's baby', with affection and indulgence, but also at times with the denigration and envy the term carries when used to refer to real mothers and real babies[3]. The creativity and leadership displayed by many of the contributors to this book exposes its practitioners, who are at once both ordinary and extraordinary human beings, to grave risk: not only the risk of failure, but the risk of their 'baby' being spoiled or damaged by envious others who would like to have conceived and developed the idea themselves. In their primary preoccupation with the development of their organizational 'baby', inventors need themselves to be nurtured by others. Too often, they are punished for leading, for daring to say 'look, here's a new direction'.

The birth of new organizational forms is threatening, for they carry within them the potential death of the old. This is why the practice model of primary care so perturbs those GPs who cleave to the practitioner model[4], and why GP fundholding continues to be resisted by some Health Authorities. This survival anxiety[5] inhibits the capacity for that constructive dialogue which alone can produce a synthesis of the two models.

The infant organizations described in this book were also asked to contain the dependency of many people: their staff, who are dependent upon them for a living, for satisfaction of a range of work motivations and career aspirations; and their patients who themselves have to learn to relate to new patterns of care, some of which may challenge previous patterns of dependency and demand.

Staff and patients identify heavily with their health care organizations. Identification has been termed the most primitive form of love and can quickly turn nasty if expectations are not met. The organizational innovator in primary care has to balance the anxieties and expectations of staff, patients, commissioning authority and wider community.

The creator of a new organizational form approaches the task with a predisposition for devotion not unlike that of a devoted parent. In order for the new creation to survive and thrive in the wider world, its creator must seek to foster in others a similar devotion or at least support, and also to ensure that his or her own devotion does not slip into exclusive possession. The new Health Authorities have a vital role to play here in supporting GP innovators.

Not only did these GPs have a vision, but they shared it with others. They also ensured that their users continued to receive quality services while they were exploring the feasibility of new organizational forms. Many chapters of this book were written in reflective mode, after conception, gestation, birth and infancy. Knowing some of the authors, I am aware that these contributions are simply the current position statements in a protracted process of documenting their organizational initiatives. Envisioning new organizational forms is not something one does purely for fun (though that is usually an ingredient). It requires to be prefaced, accompanied and followed by hard-edged thinking, writing and costing. Without these, the support required to translate vision into reality will not materialize.

Senge claims that the task of chief executives is to 'unfreeze mental models and incubate a new world view'[1]. This has been the role of creative artists, scientists and craftspeople down the ages. A group of GPs, in 1972, chose to do this when they wrote *The future general practitioner – learning and teaching*[6]. The GP contributors to the present book, however, in their role of creating new forms of primary care organization have acted more like managers than doctors. What we do not know, and urgently need to find out, is why they were able to do this.

Knowing some of them, I would judge that personal mastery is a factor. Senge described this as 'continuous clarification and deepening of personal vision, more focused use of energy, the development of patience and the capacity to see reality objectively'. What is also visible in these accounts of organizational inventiveness are the capacities, at an individual level, that Senge claims are typical of those organizations which have mastered the knack of learning from their experience. These include the capacity to:

- merge thinking and acting

- test and build prototypes

- localize

- exchange control for leverage

- exchange autonomy for accountability

- make commitment mutual

- translate invention into innovation.

While the GP contributors themselves may possess some or all of these capacities, is the translation of invention into innovation also dependent on Health Authorities and their managers possessing these capacities?

## Beyond partnership?

Some of the authors in this book, particularly Hugh Maclean in Chapter 6 and Stuart Chidgey in Chapter 12, question the capacity of partnership to deliver organizational change. Many GP partnerships are dysfunctional as groups, which is why many practices are dysfunctional as organizations, despite the best efforts of the practice manager and staff[7]. Placing practices within a multi-practice organizational context, in which certain functions, by a process of reverse delegation, are placed in a central organization, such as a multi-fund, primary care agency, or community care unit, may take the heat off inter-partner relationships within practices. Conversely, the need for a practice to be represented by one of its partners on the board of a multi-practice organization may aggravate adverse partner dynamics.

In the main, our contributors do not address the impact of new inter-practice forms of organization on partnership dynamics, and indeed what persuaded difficult partnerships to associate with these new organizations, if indeed any did so. Research is needed here.

It has been suggested that most professionals, particularly those working in partnership, are not interested in issues of organizational design[8]. This book gives the lie to that. An increasing number of GPs are now managing their practices strategically, and looking beyond them to the kind of organizational arrangements and structures described here.

What is concerning is that in a profession which now has over 50% of women in training, though fewer entering general practice as principals, there are no women GP contributors to this book. If more male than female GPs are driving primary care development, both inside the practice and beyond, as executive partners or as chairmen, chief executives, or general managers of new primary care organization, what is this saying about the place of women doctors within the primary care organizations of the future? Would a shift from partnership to company or NHS Trust forms of organization produce a different outcome?

The proliferation of multi-practice based organizations constitutes an important development in the history of practice based primary care, for while the average practice size in England and Wales is now just over four partners, in some districts over 50% of practices remain single handed. This statistic, combined with the reduction in size required to become a fundholder and the introduction of community fundholding for practices of 3000 patients means that transaction costs, between individual practices and Health Authorities, and between individual practices and providers will escalate.

Multi-practice derived organizations could transform the future structure of primary care, for while many are initially set up to address the needs of GPs as purchasers, their leaders quickly recognize that they have created an organization which can also engage in successful provider development; some multi-funds, for example, are running their own practice manager development programmes. This may be accepted more enthusiastically from a GP-owned organization than from the Health Authority. The transfer of such work needs to be marked by a corresponding transfer of resources.

The costs of organizational innovation should not be underestimated. My own consultancy involvement with a new multi-fund has illustrated the scale of the task of creating an organization from scratch. This costs money, and penetrative questions must be asked. Are new organizations tackling new work, and if so, could this be done elsewhere or in another way to similar quality standards? Are they doing work that previously was located elsewhere in the NHS? If elsewhere, then are the resources following the work, or are they doing 'old' work in new ways which results in 'added value'? And if so, to whom? The strategic shift from secondary to primary care includes the shift of managerial and administrative as well as clinical work. This too often goes unrecognized by practices, Trusts, and Commissioning Authorities.

Locality based multi-practice organizations appear to be particularly suited to those areas dominated by very small GP practices and premises, in which there is no or little likelihood that GPs will enter into partnership or form larger partnerships. The role of the new Health Authorities will be pivotal in building consensus around not only the strategic direction for primary care in its respective localities but also the organizational forms that will best serve that direction. Health Authorities whose districts reflect the full range of variation in general practice structure and culture would be wise to note the variety of organizational forms described in this book. One template alone will not address the large local let alone national variations in context.

The so-called strategic shift from secondary to primary care conveys an image of care being moved out of secondary into primary care, rather than an attempt to contain more work within the primary care setting, that is not to export it in the first place. What may be contained in a majority of practices in, for example, Oxfordshire or the South and West Region, may be contained by only a minority of practices in inner and outer London, or in east Southampton where, as David Paynton points out in Chapter 8 'a strong dependency culture is created by the local university hospital'.

More comparative research is needed on a whole range of conditions patients bring to their doctors, in order to identify those factors which predispose some practices to contain, with due regard to quality, outcome, and relative cost, work that elsewhere is exported into the secondary sector. The GP contributors to this book seek to provide as comprehensive a service as possible within their organizations, in the interests of their patients' convenience and their own work satisfaction. Not all of them practice in the leafy shires and rural settings that lie over 20 miles from the nearest district general hospital. They also welcome the responsibility of purchasing what they cannot provide, recognizing the connection between the two and the need to enhance continuity and consistency of care for their patients when they move outside the practice.

This book is a testament to the leadership capacity of its GP contributors. Are they, as has been stated of some of them, 'one-offs'? Could their organizational inventions survive their moving on? Could they be replicated reliably in their absence?

With 'its emphasis on visioning, champions, values and creation', the management literature of the 1990s has rehabilitated leadership[9]. However, 'the relationship between inspirational ideas and structures is problematic' and what Hinings *et al.* term 'loosely coupled'. It might also be said that the relationship between inspirational individuals and structures can be problematic and loosely coupled. While radical change in the way problems in health policy and health services management are construed and resolved can usually be linked to particular individuals, the development of cohesive intent and the prerequisite capacity to change individual and organizational behaviour demands the creation and implementation of new organizational frameworks and relationships the development of which must be nurtured.

General practice, however, has never had a problem with leadership. As a profession it is full of high capacity people who offer leadership at many levels but who all too frequently learn to their cost that it is not welcome. Some of the developments described here are the products of constructive followership by NHS managers of the leadership exercised by GPs. What managers will find in these pages is a wide range of organizational solutions which reflect both socio-geographic location and practice history.

## GP entrepreneurship

As small business people as well as professionals, GPs have responded readily to incentives over the years, a pattern reflected in Tom Davies' natural history of a practice in Chapter 10. Those incentives are not always purely pecuniary, but may indeed be the opportunity to wrestle with intellectual and practical challenges that are different in content, but often remarkably similar in process, to those offered by clinical work.

As owner–entrepreneurs, however, GPs may be much bolder than Health Authorities in exploring new partnerships with the private sector, particularly in relation to capital acquisition, as Stuart Chidgey details in Chapter 12. Some Health Authorities are now finding that GPs and community pharmacists are striking deals on the establishment of pharmacies inside newly built practice premises. Pharmacists are only one of many health care professionals in the semi-private and private sectors who are responding to a primary care led future. Mutuality discovered in shared business and investment strategy may well stimulate greater mutuality in formulating and implementing new clinical strategies.

While many GPs claim to be disaffected, depressed or cynical, some now recognize that when the government says its wants a primary care led NHS, at least for the moment this means GP led. Under their continued monopoly, granted by the UK system of registration and aspects of their contract, GPs are being offered a head start in setting out their stall in any future internal market in primary care. If, over the next two years, the electorate were to put 'New Labour' in government, we might be surprised to see how much of the spirit if not the letter of the NHS reforms is retained.

The inexorable rise in the capacity of modern medicine to deliver miracles and the capacity of the media to translate this into a corresponding rise in demand, together with the underlying demographic and economic features of the country now and into the 21st century, will give an incoming Labour Government little option, as John Horder demonstrates in Chapter 2, but to continue to promote a primary care led NHS. Whether this would be a GP led NHS is debatable. Paradoxically, while eschewing the internal market as such, a Labour Government might well, for example, promote and support the claims of nurses and nursing, and indeed of Community Trusts, to greater influence over the direction and management of primary care.

# UK general practice: the millennium approaches

While in the run up to the general election, there may be less debate on the desirability of a primary care led NHS, the debate on its precise shape will intensify. That debate will be less than useful if we persist in couching it in terms of what the doctor and the patient want and need, or even what GPs and patients want and need. Neither GPs nor patients are homogeneous: research suggests that what patients want and how they evaluate existing GP services differs with age, sex, socio-economic class and ethnic group. It probably also differs depending on whether they feel ill or well, and on whether they have an acute or chronic condition. So much of the debate on the ineradicable core of general practice is a kind of professional family romance. It bears little relationship to practice in areas of high population turnover, to patients who consult infrequently, and to those who are not known personally by either GP or practice staff.

Similarly, national average statistics on practice size, list size, consultation rate and achievement of contract targets are mobilized in support of certain claims, when in some areas the picture they represent would be unrecognizable.

I recently argued that general practice is in crisis[7], a crisis manifested in the person, the role, the practice and the professsion. These four manifestations are inter-related, but it is vital to understand the nature of each and of how they impact on the others. GPs continue to need 'creative assistance in integrating their image of the doctor, his patient, and the illness' with that of 'the practice, its population, and their health'[10]. Pratt[4] and the Royal College of General Practitioners in a document soon to be published on *The Nature of General Medical Practice*, begin to document this struggle. Those of us who care about general practice, though we may not be GPs ourselves, owe them the duty of responding to these attempts.

This book makes a major contribution to that debate, because it extends our concept of the practice (as organization) and therefore of general practice (as profession), and takes us beyond the practice, thereby beginning to flesh out the debate on primary managed care begun by Nichol[11].

# References

1 Senge P (1992) *The fifth discipline: the art and practice of the learning organisation.* Century Business, London.

2 Robinson B (1993) Lyme cordial. *Health Service J.* **103**: 20–22.

3 Menzies Lyth I (1975) Thoughts on the maternal role in contemporary society. In: Menzies Lyth I (ed) *Containing*

*anxiety in institutions: Selected essays.* Free Association Books, London.

4   Pratt J (1995) *Practitioners and practices: a conflict of values?* Radcliffe Medical Press, Oxford.

5   Obholzer A and Roberts V Z (eds) (1994) *The unconscious at work.* Routledge, London.

6   Royal College of General Practitioners (1972) *The future general practitioner: Learning and teaching.* British Medical Journal, for the Royal College of General Practitioners, London.

7   Huntington J (1995) *Managing the Practice: whose business?* Radcliffe Medical Press, Oxford.

8   Morris T (1992) *The end of partnership?* Paper for: Knowledge Workers in Contemporary Organizations, Lancaster.

9   Hinings C R *et al.* (1991) Change in an autonomous professional organization. *J Management Studies.* **28.**

10  Huntington J (1992) Ten years in the headlines *Health Service J.* **102**: 21.

11  Nichol D (1994) Next steps for purchasing? Population and personalised care management. In: Health Services Management Unit. *Best practice in health care commissioning*, Release 4, Churchill Livingstone, London, pp. 2.11.1–2.11.8.

# Index